Textbook of Fractures and Dislocations

Textbook of Fractures and Dislocations

Rajesh Malhotra MS
Additional Professor of Orthopaedic
All India Institute of Medical Sciences
New Delhi

PEEPEE
PUBLISHERS AND DISTRIBUTORS (P) LTD.

Textbook of Fractures and Dislocations

Published by
Pawaninder P. Vij

Peepee Publishers and Distributors (P) Ltd.
Head Office: 160, Shakti Vihar, Pitam Pura, Delhi-110 034 (India)

Corporate Office: 7/31, Ansari Road, Daryaganj, Post Box-7243
New Delhi-110002 (India)

Ph: 55195868, 9811156083

e-mail: peepee160@yahoo.co.in

e-mail: peepee160@rediffmail.com

www.peepeepub.com

First Edition: **2005**

ISBN: 81-88867-57-8

Printed at: Lordson, C-5/19, Rana Pratap Bagh, Delhi-110 007

ॐ

To

Rhythm, Ashna, Anirudh and Vrishank

You are the future

Preface

The complexity of orthopedic trauma is on the rise. At the same time, considerable advances have been made in the imaging and the treatment of fractures. Those involved with imparting the teaching and training of orthopedic trauma at the grassroot levels have an arduous task of teaching fundamentals of fracture management alongwith recently evolved paradigms. This book has been written with the aim to create a simple, concise and organized title for fracture management.The book brings together basic elements that a medical student or a general practitioner must know in order to diagnose and manage specific fractures. An insight has also been provided into newer imaging modalities, their indications and the limitations and the philosophy behind the newer methods of treatment. Abundant illustrations have been provided to make the understanding of various caveats easier. A conscious effort has been made to keep the complex classifications and controversies out of the book with the most acceptable methods of treatment receiving maximum attention.

Rajesh Malhotra

Contents

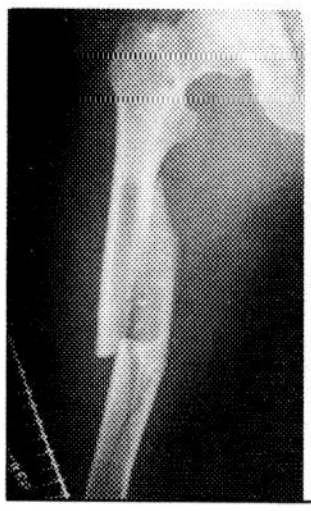

1

Introduction to Fractures

Definition, Classification, Healing, Causes of non union, Joint injuries

Definition

A fracture is a complete or incomplete break in the continuity of bone or cartilage. A fracture is usually associated with some degree of injury to the adjacent soft tissues.

A **complete** fracture is one where both cortices of the bone have broken.

An **incomplete** fracture is one where only one cortex has been broken. An incomplete fracture is relatively stable and if protected, will maintain its position indefinitely. Incomplete fractures are common in children because of the elasticity of their bones. In adults, incomplete fractures are common in short bones, flat bones and irregularly shaped bones.

Causes

Fractures are caused by:

a. **Abnormally high loads applied to normal bone** as in vehicular accidents and fall from height. These fracture are often comminuted and have more extensive soft tissue damage.
b. **Normal loads applied to abnormal bone.** These are called pathological fractures. The most common underlying condition predisposing to fracture is post menopausal osteoporosis, followed by malignancies metastatic to bone.
c. **Low levels of repetitive, unaccustomed, cyclical loading of normal bone** leading to structural fatigue. These are called stress or fatigue fractures and are commonly seen in runners. Common sties are tibia and second metatarsal.

Fracture Types

Classification of Fractures

Many terms are used to describe fractures and precise language must be used to ensure proper treatment. Fracture types can be classified according to the integrity of overlying skin, number of fragments, description of fracture lines, and the injury force applied to the bone.

i. Integrity of overlying skin and soft tissues
   a. Closed (or simple) fracture is one in which the skin and soft tissues overlying the fracture are intact and there is no communication with the outside environment.
   b. Open (or compound) fracture is one in which the fracture site communicates with the outside environment. The skin defect in these cases may be caused by the bone perforating the skin from within or by a missile of fracturing agent entering from without.
      Compound fractures are surgical emergencies because of the contamination and the possibility of infection.
ii. Number of fragments
   a. Simple fracture has a clear break and two fracture fragments. The term 'simple' is also confusingly used to described a 'closed' fracture (i.e. one which is not compound).

b. A comminuted fracture has more than two fracture fragments. There are specific types of comminuted fractures which have been given specific names because of their appearance.
   - A butterfly fragment is a wedge-shaped fragment, split off from the main fragment. On X-rays it is seen to include one cortex of the bone (Fig. 1.1).

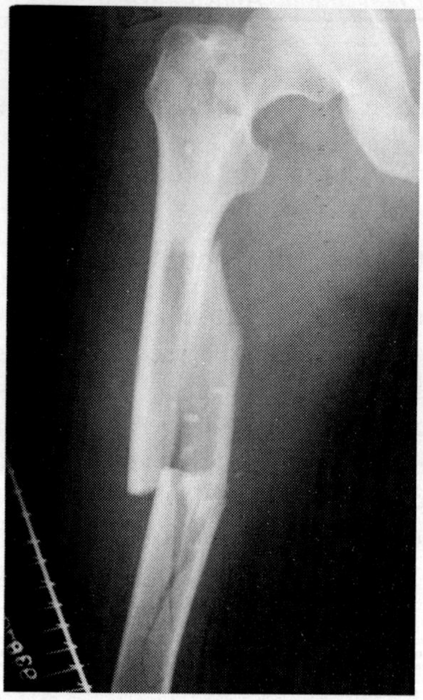

Fig. 1.1: Comminuted fracture of the femur shaft. Note the butterfly fragment on the medial side.

   - A segmental fracture is one in which the fracture divides the long bone into several segments. On X-rays the segments include both cortices of the bone (Fig. 1.2).

iii. Direction of the fractures line
   a. Transverse fracture: Fracture line is at right angles to the cortices or long axis of the bone (Fig. 1.3A). These fractures are often stable after reduction. Transverse fracture may be complete or incomplete.

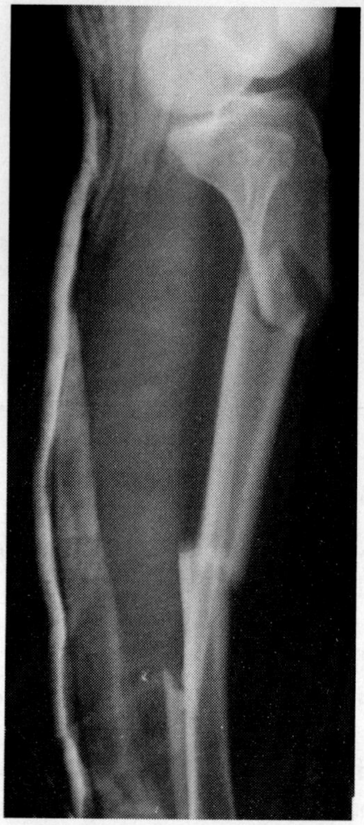

Fig. 1.2: Segmental fracture of the tibia. Note that the middle fragment includes both cortices of bone—unlike butterfly fragment

   It results from the direct injury to a long bone (*Note:* Transverse fracture of the patella is caused by an indirect injury).
   b. Oblique fracture: Fracture line runs obliquely (inclined at least 30 degrees or more) to the long axis of the bone or cortices (Fig. 1.3B). These fractures are often unstable with muscle tension leading to displacement and shortening.
   c. Spiral fracture involves a fracture line that traverses in two directions. It encircles the shaft of long bone and forms a spiral in relation to long axis and thus, spans a greater area (Fig. 1.3C). This feature often accelerates union.
   Both, the oblique and the spiral fracture, are relatively unstable and can result from a rotational force applied to the bone.

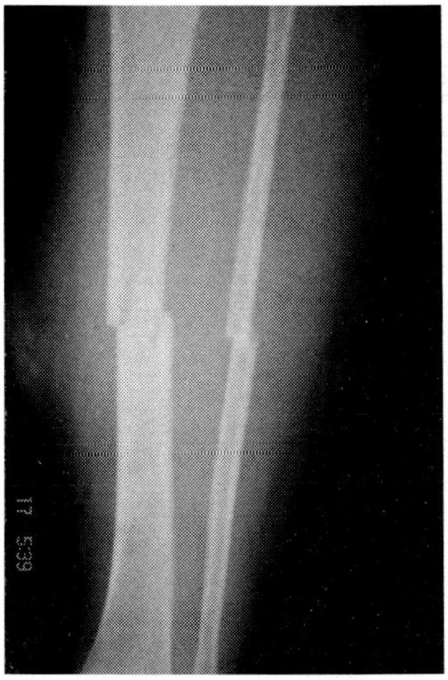

Fig. 1.3A: Transverse fracture of tibia and fibula

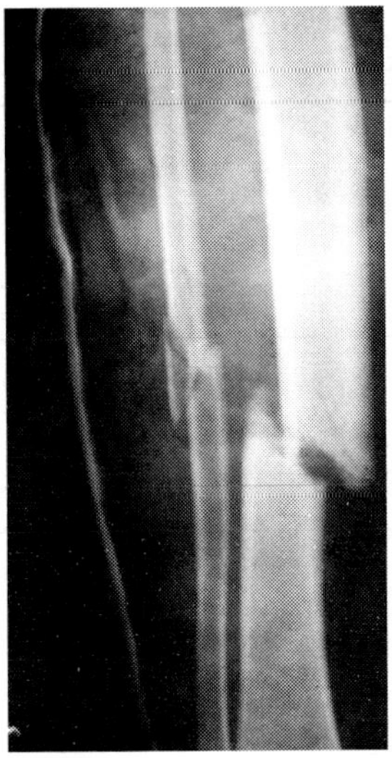

Fig. 1.3B: Oblique fracture of tibia with comminuted fracture of fibula—Note the butterfly fragment of fibula

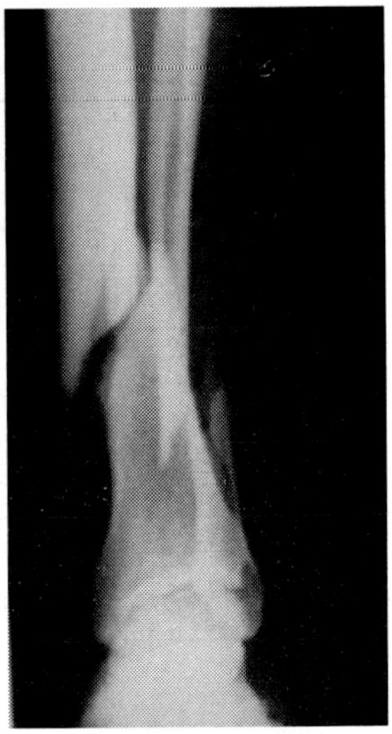

Fig. 1.3C: Spiral fracture of tibia and fibula

iv. Injury force applied to bone
   a. Impacted fracture results when a direct force is applied down the length of the bone and is characterised by telescoping of one fragment on the other. Impacted fracture usually occurs in the cancellous bone (at the ends of long bones). They are often (but not always) stable and unite rapidly.
   b. Avulsion fracture occurs after a forceful contraction of the muscle that tears its bony attachment loose (Fig. 1.4).
   c. Compression fractures occur due to axial loading in cancellous flat bones (such as vertebra, calcaneus) because they are spongy (Fig. 1.5).

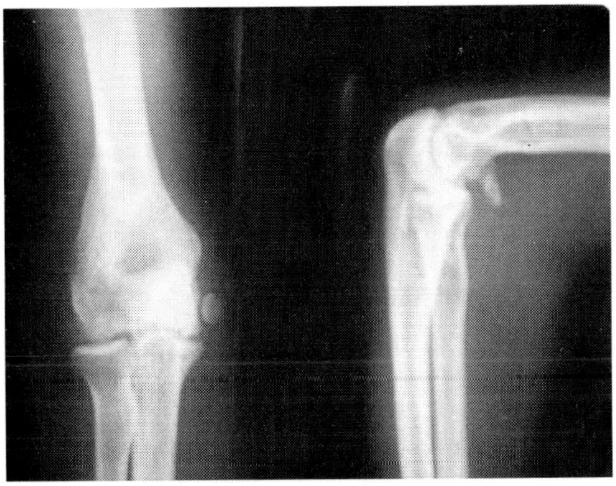

Fig. 1.4: Avulsion fracture: A valgus force to elbow causes the common flexor origin to avulse its attachment on medial epicondyle from humerus

Fracture Types in Children

Growing children have different fracture types due to unique bone qualities.

a. Greenstick fracture is fracture of only one cortex, usually in diaphysis, resulting from a bending force (Fig. 1.6).
b. Torus or buckle fracture occurs in response to compressive force and is usually seen in metaphysis (Fig. 1.7).
c. Plastic deformation occurs when the immature bone bows rather than break.

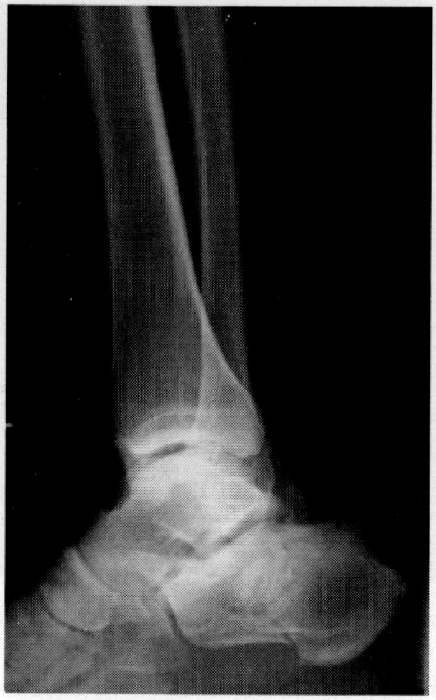

Fig. 1.5: Fracture of calcaneus. These fractures are caused by compression force—as in fall from height.

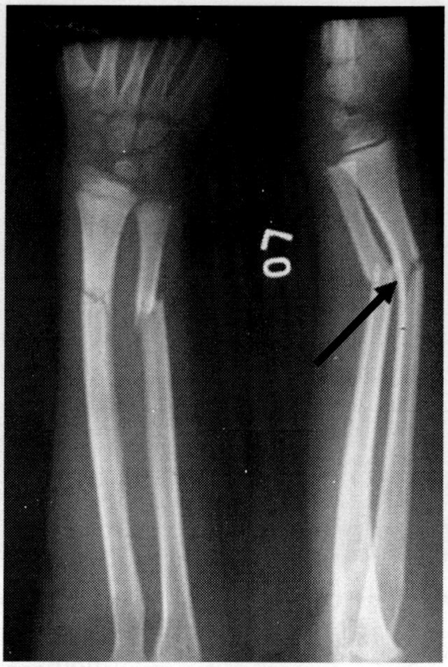

Fig. 1.6: Greenstick fracture of radius with complete fracture of ulna. Note that the dorsal cortex of radius (arrow) is intact

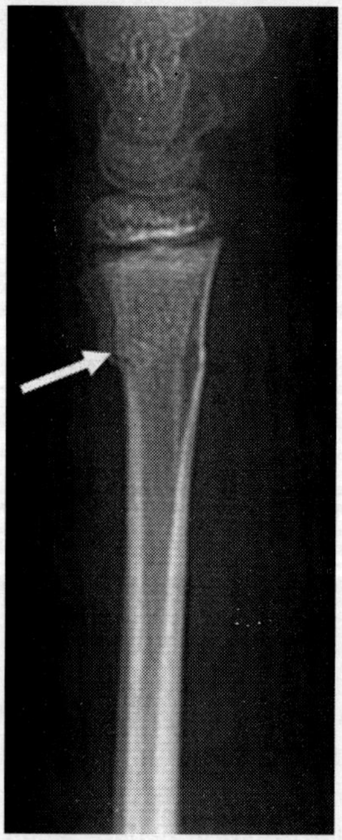

Fig. 1.7: Torus fracture of the radius. Note the buckling (arrow) of the cortex

Fracture Healing

There are three main stages of fracture healing:

1. *Inflammatory phase (starts at the time of fracture; duration 1-2 weeks):* When a bone is fractured, a hematoma from the bleeding bone ends forms around the fracture site. Hematoma is soon invaded by inflammatory cells, including neutrophils, macrophages, and phagocytes. These cells, including osteoclasts, clear necrotic tissue and prepare the ground for the reparative phase.
2. *Reparative phase (starts within 2 weeks of fracture; duration several months)*: Also called the stage of callus formation, is characterised by organization of fracture hematoma and its invasion by chondroblasts and fibroblasts that lay down matrix for callus formation. Soft callus (fibrocartilage) is composed mainly of fibrous tissue and cartilage with small amounts of bone. Osteoblasts then mineralise this soft callus, converting it into a hard callus of woven bone and increasing the stability of fracture.

3. *Remodelling phase (starts during middle of repair phase; duration months to years):* In this phase the osteoclastic and osteoblastic activities replace the immature, disorganised woven bone with a mature, organised lamellar bone which adds further stability to the fracture site. The bone is remodelled to suit function. This process allows for some correction of the angular deformities but not rotational deformities. Bone remodeling is a continuous process and is not complete until the reformation of the medullary canal and repopulation of marrow space occurs. It is dependent on the stresses that are placed on the bone.

TYPES OF BONE HEALING

Bone healing can be primary or secondary (just as the skin healing can be by primary or secondary intention) or can be also called as contact healing or callus healing respectively. Primary bone healing or contact healing occurs when there is virtually no interfragmental motion, as in an undisplaced fracture or fracture fixed by rigid fixation such as plating which does not allow micromotion between the fragments. This type of healing occurs without any evident callus.

Secondary bone healing or callus healing occurs when the bony fragments move in relation to each other. In these cases a callus forms usually within the first two weeks. The process of callus formation reduces the motion between the fragments and allows the bone to form. Nonoperative treatment and treatment with intramedullary fixation devices (such as Kuntscher's nail) allow some motion between the bone fragments and bone healing in these situations occurs with callus formation.

Factors Affecting Fracture Healing

Fracture healing may be rapid and complete or may be delayed or incomplete. A slower than usual progression of bone healing is called delayed union. An arrest or failure of healing process is called non union. When non union occurs, a pseudo-arthrosis ("Pseudo"-false, "arthrosis" joint: a false joint with pseudo capsule and synovial fluid at the site of non union—these non unions arc abnormally mobile and usually painless) or fibrous tissue forms at the site of non union. A fibrous non union may or may not be tender to palpation and may not demonstrate abnormal mobility.

The common causes of non union are:

1. ***Improper/Imperfect immobilization*** i.e. immobilization was not adequate in extent (e.g. plaster was too short) and/or duration (early discard of plaster). (*Note:* some fractures heal well even without immobilization e.g. clavicle, ribs, fibular shaft, metacarpals, metatarsals, calcaneus).
2. ***Inadequate bood supply:*** This is seen classically in the intraarticular fracture of the neck of the femur and the waist or proximal third fractures of scaphoid. Inadequate blood supply in the lower third of tibia and distal third of ulna, due to sparse soft tissue attachments which bring vascularity with them, commonly leads to delayed union or non union.
3. ***Intraarticular fractures:*** Intraarticular fractures often have healing problems as:
   a. synovial fluid washes away the fracture hematoma.
   b. synovial fluid collagenases weaken the fracture callus.
   c. there may be excessive motion between the fracture fragments.
   d. Smaller size of fracture fragment(s) provides inadequate/insufficient purchase to fixation devices (screws, pins etc.).
4. ***Inadequate contact between the bony fragments:*** This can be due to:
   a. Improper reduction leading to complete off-ending of fracture fragments.
   b. Interposition of soft tissues between the bony fragments.
   c. Excessive distraction at fracture site e.g. due to:
      i. Weight of the plaster as in the case of hanging cast given for fracture humerus

leading to loss of contact at the fracture site.

ii. Excessive traction as excessive weight on the upper tibial pin traction leading to distraction at the femoral shaft fracture site.

d. Bone loss as in a compound fracture.

e. Avulsion fractures: The bony fragment attached to the muscle-tendon unit is displaced away from the bed and will not heal unless reduced back and fixed operatively.

f. Comminuted and segmental fractures caused by high velocity injuries (*Note:* Comminuted fractures caused by low impact trauma heal rapidly as they provide large surface area for union and the soft tissue attachments are often intact).

g. Due to stabilizing device: After fracture the bone ends undergo necrosis due to loss of blood supply. When these necrotic ends are resorbed, a gap may appear which may be maintained by fixation device such as external fixator or a nail leading to non union.

5. *Infection.*
6. *Injury to soft tissues.*

Severe injuries are associated with significant injury to the soft tissues and lead to delayed or non union. Injury to overlying skin (as in compound fractures) leads to loss of fracture hematoma and injury to muscles and periosteum compromises vascularity.

More than one of these factors may combine to thwart union in a fracture. *For example:* A fracture of distal one third of the tibia often undergoes delayed or non union because:

i. It has poor blood supply due to sparse soft tissue attachments.

ii. It is subcutaneous and the fracture spike or the injury may violate the overlying skin leading to:

a. Loss of fracture hematoma
b. Risk of osteomyelitis
c. Loss of bony fragment at the accident site through the wound

iii. These are often high velocity injuries in young patients and may be associated with disruption of soft tissues, further compromising the vascularity of the fracture fragments.

iv. Associated soft tissue injury may necessitate treatment using external fixator which may contribute to delayed or non union.

Note: Fracture through a diseased bone for example due to infection or malignancy (Fig. 1.8) also result in non union.

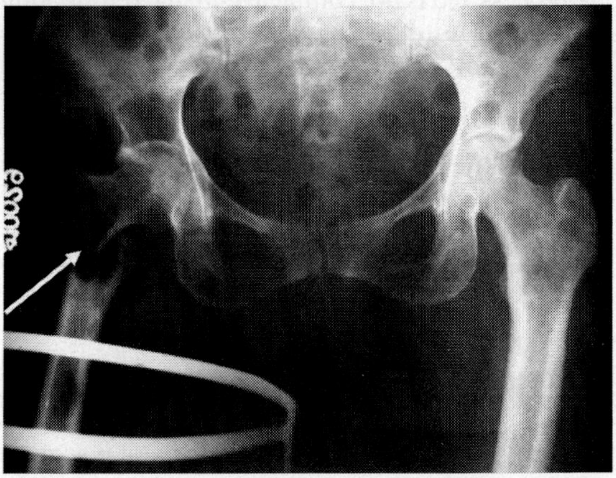

Fig. 1.8: Pathological fracture through an area of destruction in the right upper femur (arrow). The patient was suffering from multiple myeloma. Such fractures are prone to non union

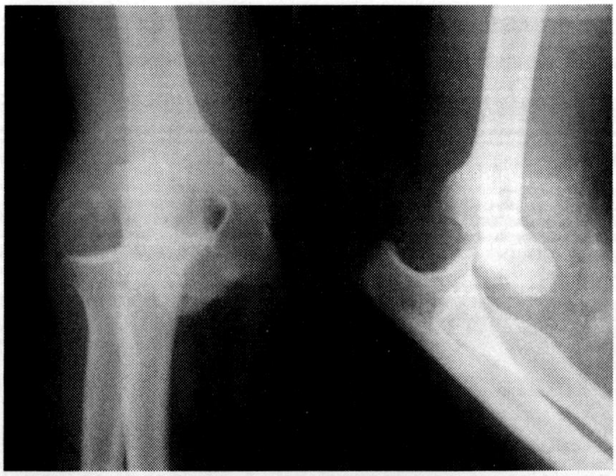

Fig. 1.9: Dislocation of the elbow. Note the complete loss of contact between the lower humerus, and, radius and ulna

JOINT INJURIES

Dislocations and subluxations occur when there is complete or partial loss of contact between the two opposing articular surfaces of the joint respectively (Fig. 1.9). Dislocation of a joint may or may not appear in conjunction with a fracture of bone. In dislocation, the soft tissues such as the joint capsule and ligaments are torn and the blood vessels supplying the metaphyses of bone which enter through the soft tissues near the joint are often stretched or torn.

A fracture dislocation is present when a joint has dislocated and there is, in addition, a fracture of a related bony components.

A dislocation is a dire emergency when

a. There is an interruption of vascularity due to dislocation with risk of avascular necrosis (as in dislocation of hip which can result in avascular necrosis of the femoral head; dislocation of talus, or, dislocation of the lunate).

b. When there is stretching of the overlying skin due to dislocation with the risk of necrosis and sloughing of overlying skin (as in the casc of complete dislocation of talus).

c. Open or compound dislocation when there is a possibility of infection.

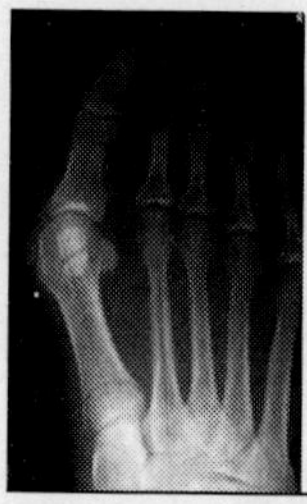

2 Evaluation of Musculoskeletal Trauma

Diagnosis, Neurovascular injuries, Imaging, Evaluation of old fractures

The spectrum of musculoskeletal injuries varies from life threatening, polytrauma injury to bruises or torn ligaments caused by simple falls. The diagnosis of a fracture or dislocation is relatively obvious (Table 2.1). The key is not to miss an associated injury.

Table 2.1: Diagnosis of fractures

Symptoms	*Signs*
Pain	Deformity
Swelling	Tenderness
Bruising	Swelling at fracture site
Inability to use the limb	Bruising around fracture
	Abnormal mobility*
	Crepitus **(should not be elicited)** on movement of fragments*
	Loss of transmitted movements*
	Impairment of function

*Provide conclusive evidence

A history is obtained and physical examination performed on all patients who have sustained a fracture or dislocation. A focussed history is obtained about when, where and how the injury occurred, presence of associated injuries and previous injuries of the affected region. Severe and unremitting pain (especially at a site away from the location of fracture as established by examination and X-ray) may indicate a compartment syndrome (see page 41-42) and high index of suspicion should be maintained to diagnose this catastrophic complication. A past medical history is obtained to determine whether there are pre existing conditions that alter the choice of management (as, for example, a recent myocardial infarction may preclude surgical treatment of the fracture, or, if the function of that extremity was already compromised by preexisting injury or disease). Hand dominance and occupation are important facts to elicit in history. A social history provides clues regarding the use of alcohol, tobacco and drugs. History of allergies may be important to determine the choice of drugs for the patient.

The initial examination should quickly assess the vitals and the consciousness. Certain fractures can lead to considerable blood loss and result in hypovolaemia and even shock (Table 2.2). Further examination includes evaluating the neurovascular status, inspection for deformity and breaks in the skin (Fig. 2.1), and, assessment of the soft tissue injury. Presence of a severe bruise on the forehead after a car accident may suggest the possibility of the whiplash injury to the cervical spine even if the patient may not initially complain of the neck pain. Palpation for areas of maximum tenderness allows the determination of exact fracture site and to order appropriate X-rays.

Active and passive range of motion of surrounding joints is assessed. The circulation is

Table 2.2: Estimated blood loss (internal bleeding) in the fracture hematoma in various fractures

Fracture	**Average Blood loss (ml)**
Pelvis	1500-3000
Femur	1500
Tibia and fibula	500
Humerus	250
Radius and ulna	150-250

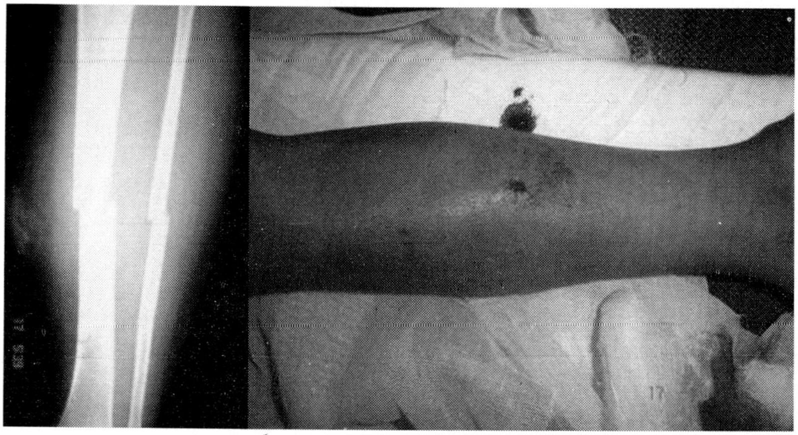

Fig. 2.1: Compound fracture of both bones of the leg. X-rays (left) show marked swelling indicating severe injury to soft tissues. Leg (right) showed breach of skin

assessed by palpating pulses, looking for capillary refill in the nail bed and by color of the skin. Table 2.3 indicates the site of palpation of peripheral pulses. Soft tissues in case of extremity fractures and/or vascular injuries in the extremities should be carefully palpated to rule out the existence of the compartment syndrome when they become swollen and tense. There is impairment of 2-point discrimination and pain on passive stretching of the digits. It should be remembered that the peripheral pulses may be present even in advanced compartment syndrome. Measurement of the compartment pressure is indicated if compartment syndrome is suspected.The detailed neurologic examination is done including sensory and motor system and special tests for the peripheral nerve injuries. The neurovascular injuries are commonly associated with some fracture patterns (Tables 2.4 and 2.5). High velocity injuries with severe injury to soft tissues and comminution of bones may be associated with vascular injuries (Fig. 2.2). A complete physical examination of cardiovascular, respiratory, gastrointestinal, genitourinary and neurologic systems must be performed in all cases.

Table 2.3: Palpation of peripheral pulses

Peripheral pulse	*Location*
Femoral artery	Femoral triangle
Popliteal artery	Popliteal fossa
Posterior tibial	Behind medial malleolus
Dorsalis pedis	Lateral to base of the first metatarsal
Brachial artery	Cubital fossa
Radial artery	Lateral to flexor carpi radialis tendon
Ulnar artery	Lateral to flexor carpi ulnaris tendon

Table 2.4: Fracture(s)/Dislocation(s) commonly associated with nerve injuries

Fracture/Dislocation	*Nerve injured*
Shoulder dislocation	Axillary nerve, brachial plexus
Humerus	Radial nerve injury
Supracondylar humerus	Radial > median > ulnar
Radial head dislocation	Posterior interosseous nerve
Elbow dislocation	Median > ulnar
Hip dislocation (posterior)	Sciatic nerve
Knee dislocation	Common peroneal nerve
Fibular neck fracture	Common peroneal nerve
Unstable spine injuries	Spinal cord/cauda equina

The area of injury, joint distal to the injury and one joint proximal to the injury should be carefully examined.

Table 2.5: Fracture(s)/Dislocation(s) commonly associated with arterial injuries

Fracture/Dislocation	*Arterial injury*
Shoulder dislocation	Axillary artery
Supracondylar humerus fracture	Brachial artery
Elbow dislocation	Brachial artery
Fracture shaft femur (Proximal 1/3rd)	Profunda femoris
Knee dislocation	Popliteal artery
Displaced fractures of proximal 1/3rd tibia	Popliteal artery

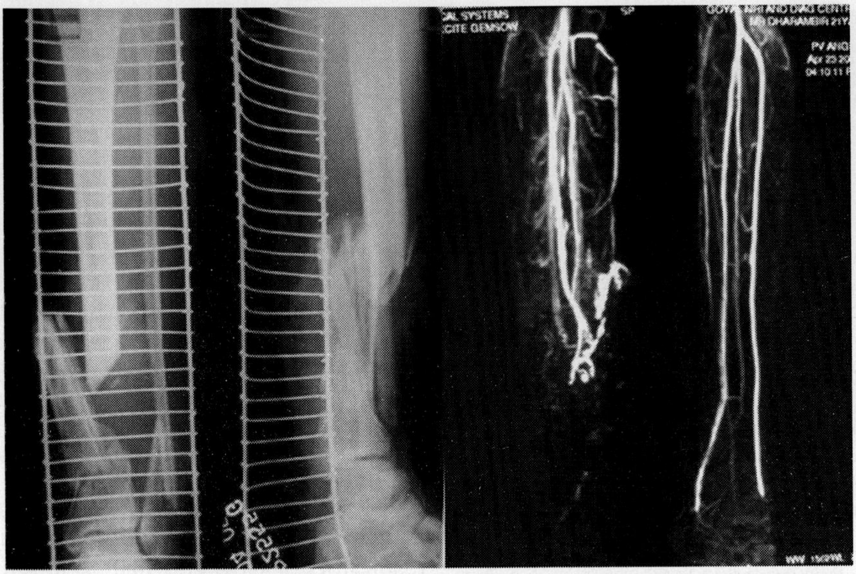

Fig. 2.2: Comminuted fracture of both bones of the leg with severe injury to soft tissues and absent distal circulation. Angiography (right) showed vascular injury. Note: Compare the vascular outline with intact vessels in uninjured limb (extreme right)

Certain mechanisms give rise to a combination of injuries to different regions of the body e.g. presence of fracture of dorsolumbar spine following a fall from height should raise the suspicion of bilateral calcaneus fractures. Table 2.6 provides a list of such related injuries which share a common mechanism.

Table 2.6: Commonly associated fractures with similar mechanism of injury

Diagnosed injury	*Look for*	*Remark*
Knee	Hip, Spine	Dash board injury
Wrist	Elbow	Essex Lopresti
Skull	Cervical spine	Vehicular accident Unconscious patient
Calcaneus	Knee, dorso-lumbar spine	Fall from height

X-ray

A. Principles of obtaining X-rays in a patient with musculoskeletal injury
   1. Splint the injured part whenever possible to provide pain relief and prevent additional injury to adjacent structures
   2. Always obtain at least two views at right angles to each other (e.g. anteroposterior and lateral views most commonly)
   3. X-rays should include the entire bone and any adjacent bone or joint that has significant tenderness
   4. X-ray opposite, noninjured extremity (in children) if an unfused epiphysis appears like a fracture but clinically the region is not tender. Table 2.7 elaborates common normal variations which are often mistaken as fractures
   5. Take additional X-rays (special views or at a later date) if the physical examination strongly suggests a fracture but initial X-rays are normal. For example, oblique views are often needed to diagnose the fracture of scaphoid but if the initial X-rays are normal, yet the suspicion of the fracture is strong, X-rays are repeated after two weeks of plaster immobilisation when the fracture line may be apparent due to resorption of bone at the fracture site

Table 2.7: Radiological variants mistaken as fractures

1. Accessory bones	Separate centres of ossification adjacent to parent bone. **Most common in foot (Fig. 2.3).** These have smooth rounded border surrounded by cortical bone, often bilateral
2. Epiphyses	Especially in hand, olecranon, base of 5th metatarsal; take opposite side X-rays
3. Juxta articular calcification	Calcification at insertion of tendons. Amorphous; no trabeculae
4. Multipartite conditions	Bi- or Tri-partite patella (Fig. 2.4), bipartite scaphoid; usually bilateral, line of separation curved with smooth, dense apposing surfaces
5. Neural foramina	Esp. large foramina in young bones. Smooth oblique appearance
6. Pseudofracture (umbauzonen) (Looser zones)	Seen in Osteomalacia (Fig. 2.5), Milkman syndrome, Rickets, Paget's disesae. Incomplete, transverse lucent zones, bilateral, no h/o trauma
7. Sesamoids	Bones that develop in tendon and occur near a joint. Commonly seen in foot (Fig. 2.6), hand

B. Approach to evaluation of X-rays for skeletal injury
1. First check whether you have all the views necessary to evaluate the fracture and whether they are marked right (R) or left (L) in agreement with clinically injured extremity.
2. Look at soft tissues for swelling, muscle planes (delineated by fat between planes) and presence of air (Fig. 2.7) (as in compound fractures or in cases with gas gangrene). A displaced soft tissue shadow may suggest

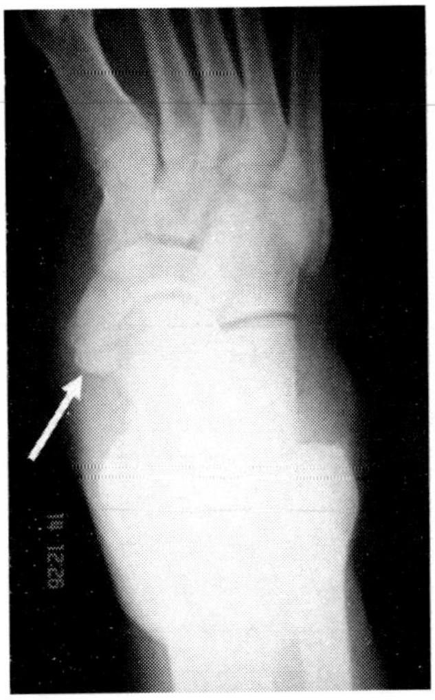

Fig. 2.3: Accessory navicular (arrow)

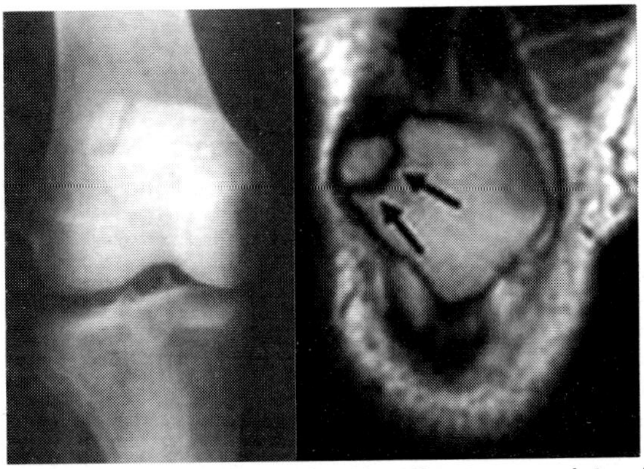

Fig. 2.4: Bipartite patella: Usually at superolateral pole, usually bilateral, rounded margin with smooth, dense apposing surfaces (arrows)

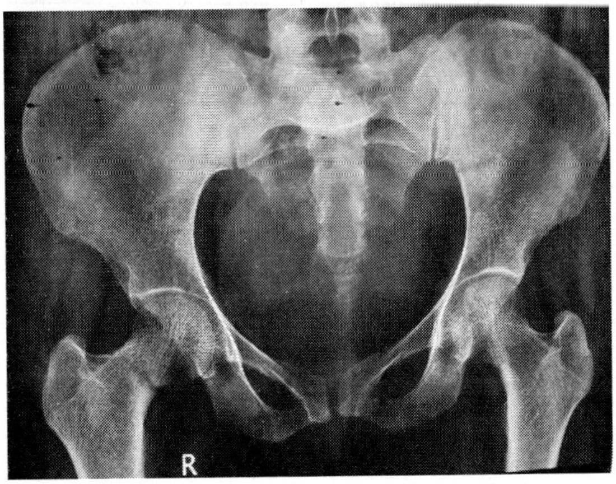

Fig. 2.5: Looser zones in osteo malacia

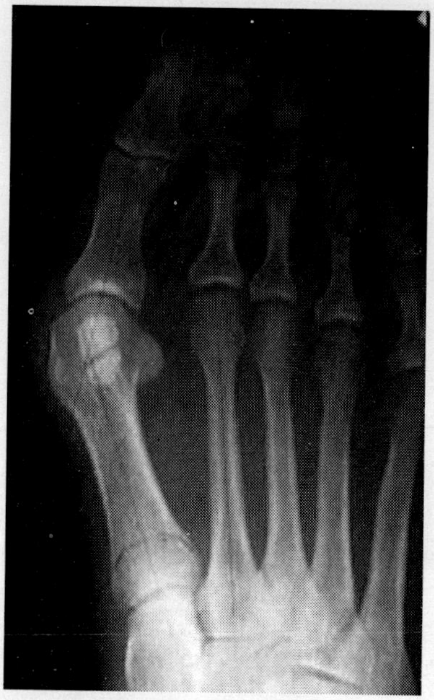

Fig. 2.6: Sesamoids in relation to big toe. This patient also has hallux valgus

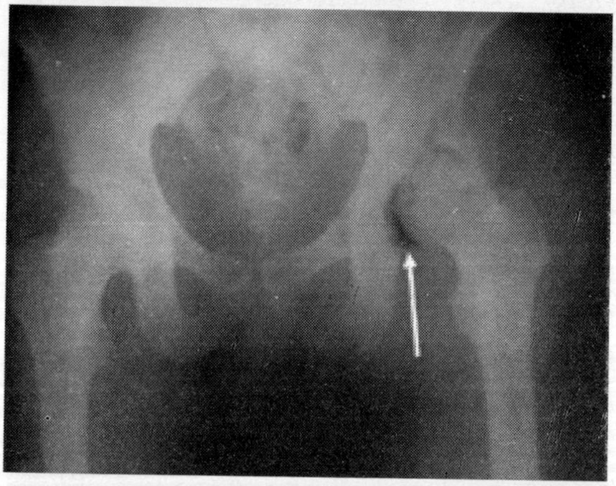

Fig. 2.7: Air in the hip joint (arrow). Patient had a compound fracture dislocation of the left hip joint

the presence of an undisplaced fracture which might not be obvious on the X-rays e.g.

a. An anterior (coronoid) or posterior (olecranon) fat pad sign may suggest a supracondylar fracture of humerus (Fig. 8.2).

b. Presence of lucent fat droplets in the knee suggests intra-articular fracture.

3. Assess the bone
   a. Bone involved—which bone is involved? It is normal or the fracture has occurred through the localized disease of bone (pathological fracture)? Is the bone abnormal suggestive of existence of a generalised bone disease? Does the fracture appear to be recent or old? If it is old, what is the status of the union?
   b. Location of the fracture
      - Diaphyseal, metaphyseal, articular (extending to joint surface) or physeal (affecting growth plate in children)
      - Location within a bone can also be described as proximal (proximal third, proximal fourth etc.) or distal and as fracture involving the anatomically distinct area within the bone as head, neck, shaft or base
   c. Type of fracture
      - Simple or comminuted
      - Transverse, oblique or spiral
   d. Displacement of the fracture
      Displacements are described according to the following rules
      i. All displacements are described with relation to the distal fragment i.e. medial displacement means the distal fragment has displaced medially.
      ii. Angulation and tilt are two distinct terms which are not interchangeable (Fig. 2.8).
         - **Angulation** is described in relation to the shaft (diaphyseal) fractures where the two fragments are not parallel or colinear. Angulation may be in coronal plane (varus, valgus) or the sagittal plane (procurvatum or recurvatum). Angulation is

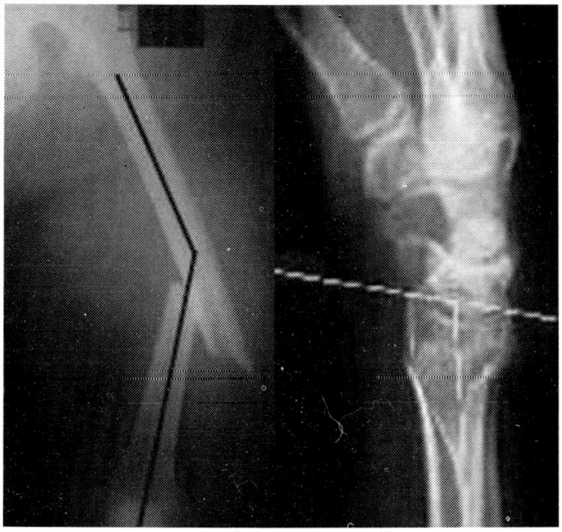

Fig. 2.8: Angulation versus tilt. Femoral shaft fracture on the left has lateral angulation on AP view. Colles' fracture on the right has dorsal tilt on the lateral view

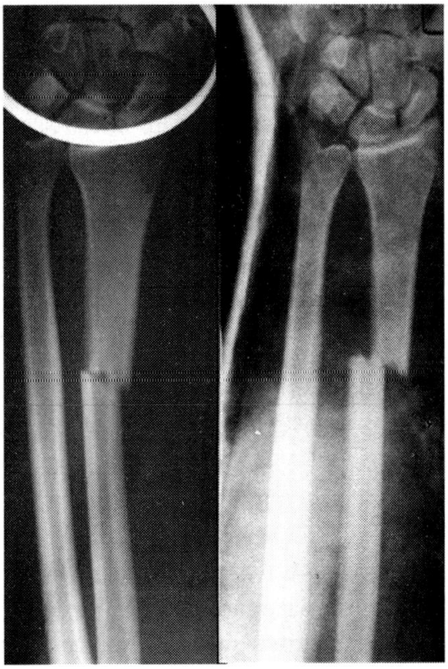

Fig. 2.9: Bony contact. X-ray on the left has more than 90 percent contact between fragments. At a later date the fracture displaced and now showed only one third contact

said to exist to the side to which the apex of the angle points.

Note the degree of angulation e.g. there is 30°medial angulation.

Tilt is described in relation to the metaphyseal fractures which are close to the joint. Tilt is said to exist to the side to which the adjacent articular surface of the distal fragment faces.

iii. The displacements in a fracture can be:
- Shortening or proximal migration when there is over-riding or impaction of the fragments.
- Translation or displacement which results in reduced contact between the bony fragments (Fig. 2.9). In most severe cases there is complete loss of bony contact; more commonly, some apposition remains and this may be described as a percentage of the fracture surface e.g. there is 40% bony contact.
- Angulation: care should be taken to avoid confusion between the angulation and tilt. An anterior angulation will tilt the distal articular surface posteriorly.
- Rotation: One fragment rotates in its long axis in relation to the other. This rotational or torsional deformity may be due to internal or the external rotation of the distal fragment. It may not be obvious in routine X-rays but is important to recognise as it can cause serious functional limitations, especially in the upper extremity. Malrotation is suspected in:

(a) Single bone fractures by difference in the diameter of the fracture fragments at the fracture site. Also, the profile of the fragments may appear different—an AP of proximal joint may show distal joint in lateral view.

(b) In two bone fractures (forearm, legs) as difference in the interosseous space between the proximal and the distal fracture fragments at the fracture site.

iv. Think whether the deformity or displacement is explained by the soft tissue attachments/deforming forces on the fracture fragment(s). For example, in case of a femoral shaft fracture, proximal fragment is abducted due to the pull of abductor muscles. However, adduction of the proximal fragment is pathognomonic of an associated posterior dislocation of the ipsilateral hip which may have been missed.

e. Look at each joint: Is the joint normal or degenerated or arthritic? Has the fracture involved the joint? Is the joint surface smooth or has areas of depression?

f. Evaluate need for further imaging studies as tomograms, CT scan, MRI, or Bone scan.

* Tomograms: are often required for cervical spine trauma or complex intra-articular fractures where depression of some of the articular fragments is suspected. Tomograms have largely been replaced by computed tomography in current practice.

* CT scan is indicated:
- In the fractures or fracture-dislocations of the spine to demonstrate retropulsion of fragments (see BURST FRACTURES Page 53-54) and compromise of the neural canal.
- To diagnose a fracture when it is not revealed on plain X-rays-especially carpal bones.
- To evaluate comminuted intra articular fractures (calcaneus, tibial plateau, acetabulum, distal radius) where it can diagnose depressed articular fragments and also for planning reconstruction (by 3-D reconstructions) (Fig. 2.10).
- To diagnose union as in case of scaphoid fracture.

* MRI is indicated for:
- Evaluation of spinal cord in spinal injuries
- Diagnosis of ligament injuries (especially within the knee)
- Diagnosis of fracture (e.g. scaphoid fracture)
- Evaluation of vascularity (e.g. vascularity of femoral head following the intra capsular fracture of the femoral neck) (Fig. 2.11).

* Bone scan is indicated for:
- Diagnosis of fracture not evident on plain X-rays e.g. scaphoid fracture
- To assess union of a fracture
- To assess complications of fracture/treatment:
  a. Avascular necrosis of the femoral head following the fracture neck of femur

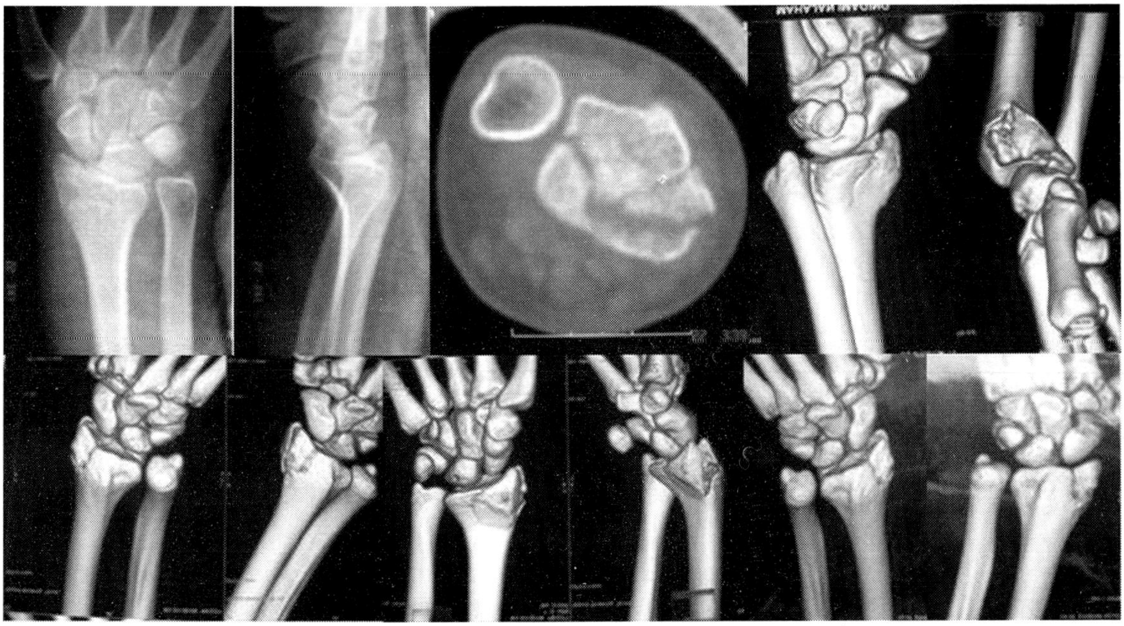

Fig. 2.10: CT scan is especially useful for evaluation of complex intraarticular fractures. The bony fragment and comminution is not very well appreciated on X-rays (Top left). Axial cuts on CT scan (Top middle) show comminution. 3D reconstruction images (Top right and bottom) can show the comminution, size, number and displacement of fragments especially depressed ones

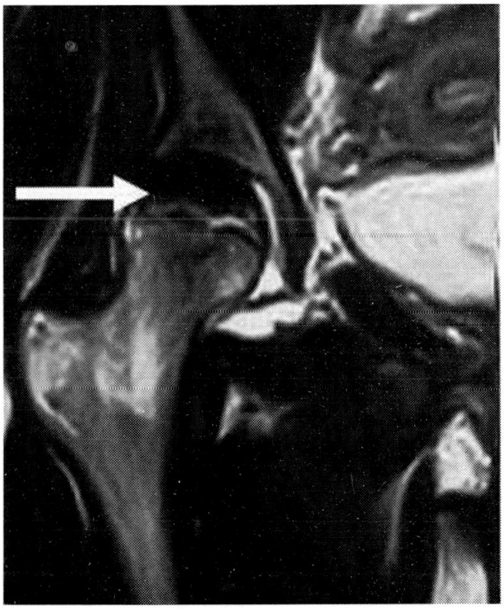

Fig. 2.11: MRI showing avascular necrosis of femoral head (arrow) MRI is the most reliable investigation for early and accurate diagnosis of avascular necrosis

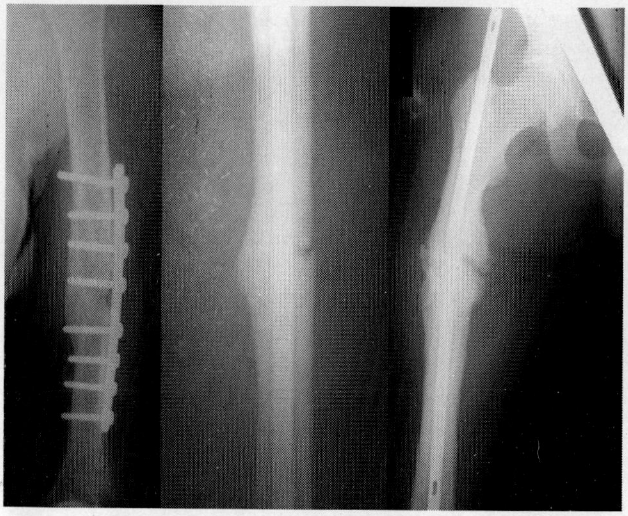

Fig. 2.12: Assessment of fracture healing. (i) Left: Healed fracture. No fracture line seen. Cortical continuity; (ii) Middle: Healing fracture. Fracture line partly seen. Partial cortical continuity; (iii) Right: Failure of healing. Hypertrophic non union. Exuberant callus but not bridging, sclerosed and smoothened bone ends. Fracture line visible. Note that the intramedullary nail is very short and this possibly lead to non union due to inadequate splintage.

b. Diagnosis of complications as (i) infection after internal fixation, and (ii) Reflex sympathetic dystrophy following the injury or treatment.

EVALUATION OF OLD FRACTURES

If a fracture is not recent, it is important to evaluate whether the healing (union) has started, is progressing or has stopped/failed (Fig. 2.12).

When a fracture is healing, there may be tenderness and/or mobility at the fracture site and the X-rays show evidence of callus formation without evidence of solid union or non union (failure of union). The clinical and radiological features of uniting, united and ununited fractures are shown in Table 2.8.

Table 2.8: Clinical and Radiological assessment of bony union

Status of union	*Clinical*			*Radiological*			
	Pain	*Tenderness*	*Abnormal mobility*	*Callus*		*Trabeculae*	*Other features*
				Bridging	*Non bridging*		
Healing fracture	+	+	+		+	No continuity	Fracture lines not distinct; some osteoporosis
Healed fracture (united)	—	—	—	++	—	Continuity	Fracture line not visible or sometimes (partially) visible
Failure of healing (Non union)	±	±	+ usually except fibrous union	—	May be present (hypertrophic) or absent (atrophic)	No continuity	Fracture line visible; fracture ends smooth and sclerosed; osteoporosis may be present

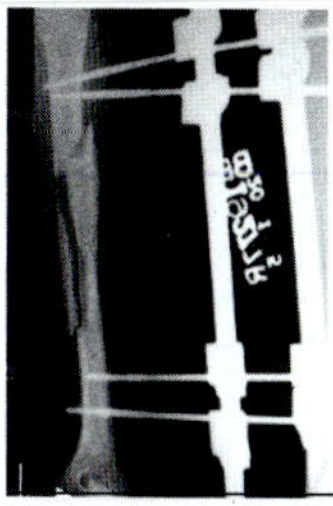

3 Principles of Treatment of Fractures

Initial Assessment, Selection of Definitive Treatment, Fractures in children

The initial assessment of a fracture must answer some important questions (Table 3.1). In a multiply injured patient following measures are mandatory for resuscitation:

a. Secure adequate airway.
   - Neck should not be moved during airway management to prevent damage from an unrecognized neck injury.
   - Open the mouth and inspect. Clear it of loose bodies, broken teeth etc.
   - Lift the chin, insert nasal airway; Intubate if the patient is unable to protect the airway.
   - If unable to secure upper airway (bleeding in oral cavity, fracture mandible), (Fig. 3.1) perform immediate cricothyroidotomy.

Table 3.1: Initial assessment of injured patient

1.	Is the patient stable vitally? Airway, Bleeding, Circulation Proceed further only if the answer to question is yes
2.	Are there any associated injuries to: • Vessels, viscera, skin, nerves? • The same extremity or elsewhere in the skeleton?
3.	Is the fracture stable or unstable? Unstable fracture can cause injury to spinal cord (unstable spinal fracture) or the soft tissues (skin, nerves, vessels) and must be splinted/immobilized by some form of splintage/traction before transport

b. Ensure that the patient is breathing. If not:
   - Ventilate with AMBU bag and mask, send arterial blood for blood gases analysis.
   - Decreased oxygenation occurs due to pneumothorax (Fig. 3.2) (other features are deviation of trachea to opposite side, absent breath sounds, tympanitic percussion note, distended neck veins, open sucking wound), Hemothorax (Fig. 3.3) (trachea deviated to opposite side, absent breath sounds, dull percussion note) or a flail chest (Fig. 3.4) (paradoxical motion of chest, crepitus on palpation due to fractured ribs). Hemothorax needs to be drained (by

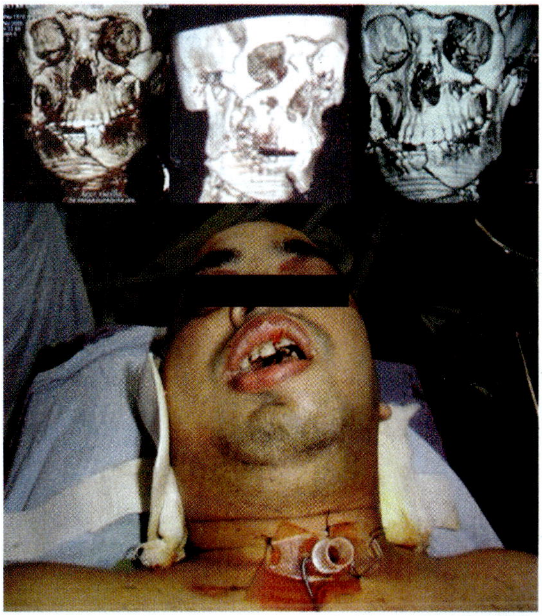

Fig. 3.1: CT scan with 3D reconstruction in a polytrauma patient with multiple fractures in facial skeleton. Facial injuries (especially fractures of mandible) may lead to obstruction of the airway and may become life threatening. Bottom: A tracheostomy in such cases secures the patient's airway

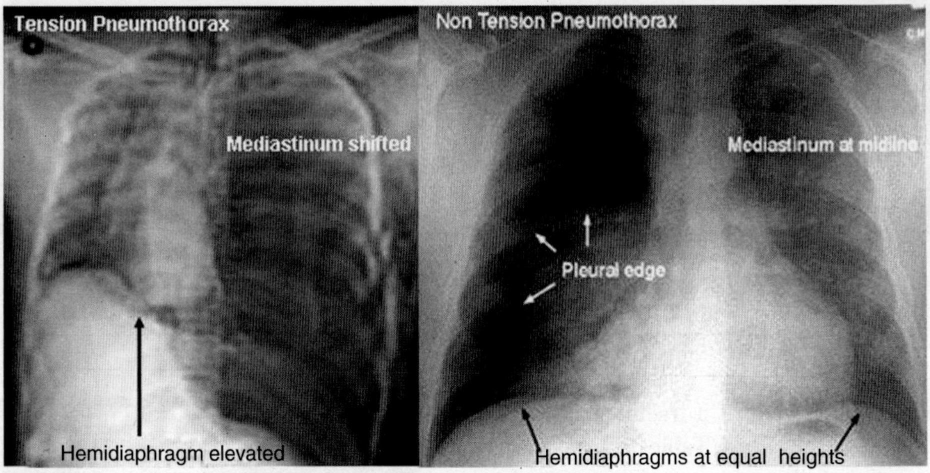

Fig. 3.2: Tension pneumothorax (left) and non tension pneumothorax (right). Note the difference in mediastinal shift and level of hemidiaphragm

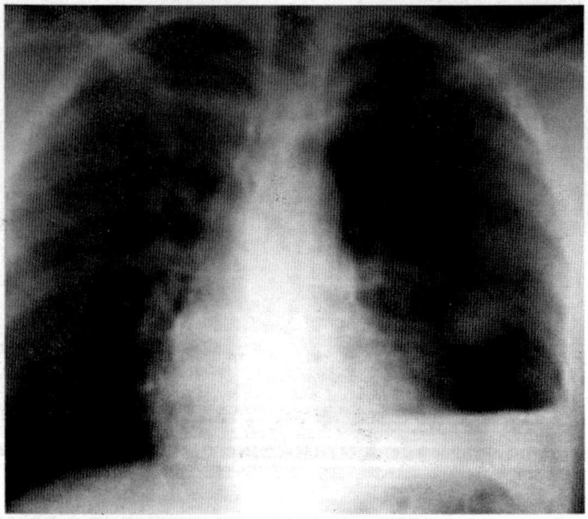

Fig. 3.3: Left hemothorax

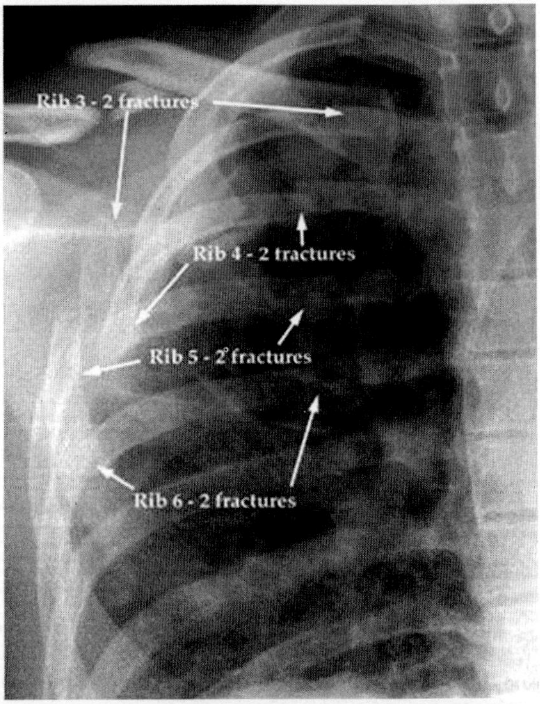

Fig. 3.4: Flail chest

intracostal drainage) while the pneumothorax is managed by inserting a large-bore needle into the mid-clavicular line at the second intercostal space. It is replaced by chest tube once the patient is stabilized. Occlusive dressing is applied for open pneumothorax but the dressing should not be taped on one side to allow the air to escape. It is followed by surgical wound closure and a chest tube. Flail chest is managed by positive pressure ventilation (Positive End-Expiratory Pressure: PEEP).

c. Assess circulation by pulse, blood pressure and peripheral circulation (capillary refill, peripheral pulses). In trauma patients shock is hemorrhagic until proved otherwise. **Shock in a traumatised patient should never be attributed to head injury**. Potential third space blood loss in closed injuries can give rise to shock (Table 3.2).

Table 3.2: Potential third space blood loss in closed injuries

Injured site	*Potential blood loss (internal hematoma)*
Chest	3000 ml/side
Abdomen	Variable
Retroperitoneum	3000 ml
Pelvis	1500-3000 ml
Extremity fracture	
Femur	1500 ml
Humerus/Tibia	500 ml

In case of inadequate circulation suggesting shock:

- Control external bleeding by applying sterile dressing and direct pressure.
- Insert two large-bore lines (14G), take samples for blood group typing and cross matching and infuse 2 litres Ringer Lactate while the blood is awaited. 'O' negative blood is used for life threatening emergencies. Injured extremity should be avoided for vascular access. Saphenous vein cutdown in adults or intraosseous (Tibia) infusions for children younger than 6 years may be used.
- Serially monitor blood pressure and urine out put and preferably place central venous line. Serial hematocrit monitoring should be undertaken to replace blood as indicated till patient is hemodynamically stable.
- Unstable extremity fractures should be splinted or immobilised in traction to limit haemorrhage. Patients with unstable pelvis fracture should not be repeatedly shifted or moved as it may lead to more internal bleeding.
- Diagnostic peritoneal lavage, FAST (Focussed Assessment with Sonography for Trauma), CT, MRI or angiography (with or without embolization) or immediate operative intervention may be indicated for the diagnosis and control of the cause of hemorrhage.
- Military antishock trouser (MAST) can be used to increase peripheral resistance, decrease lower extremity blood pooling, immobilize lower extremity fracture and decrease intrapelvic volume in cases with displaced pelvic fractures. It is simple, rapid and reversible but limits the access to abdomen, pelvis and extremities and can result in compartment syndrome or exacerbation of congestive heart failure. *Note:* In patient with thoracic cord injury due to spine injury, sympathetic disruption may lead to inability to maintain vascular tone. These patients have hypotension without tachycardia or vasoconstriction which does not respond to fluid resuscitation. Fluid overload should be avoided in these patients and vasoactive drugs are needed after volume restoration.

d. Neurologic assessment is done initially by level of consciousness, pupillary response, sensation and motor response in all the extremities, and, rectal tone and sensation. Glasgow Coma Scale (Table 3.3) can assess brain damage and potential recovery by measuring three behavioural responses: eye opening, best verbal response and best motor response.

Note: Patients with GCS < 13, systolic BP < 90 and respiratory rate > 29 or < 10/min should be referred to trauma centre as they need detailed investigations for adequate evaluation of injuries. After finishing initial clinical evaluation, the fracture (s) should be splinted.

Emergency splinting performs three functions:

1. Prevents further soft tissues injury by fracture fragments
2. Relieves pain, and,
3. Lowers the incidence of clinical fat embolism.

Table 3.3: Glasgow Coma Scale (GCS)

Response	*Score*
A. Eye opening (E)	
1. Spontaneous	4
2. in response to verbal command	3
3. in response to pain	2
4. No	1
B. Best motor response (M)	
1. Obeys commands	6
2. Localises stimulus	5
3. Withdraws to stimulus	4
4. Flexor response	3
5. Extensor response	2
6. None	1
C. Verbal response (V)	
1. Oriented	5
2. Confused conversation	4
3. Inappropriate words	3
4. Incomprehensible phonation	2
5. None	1

The range of GCS score (E + M+ V) is 3-15.

When applying a splint or shifting a patient with fracture, the pain is reduced if traction is applied to the limb. The upper extremity fractures are immobilised by Cramer wire splints while the proximal femoral and femoral shaft fractures are best immobilised in a Thomas splint. Temporary immobilisation of upper extremity fractures can be provided by wearing the shirt or jacket over the extremity with the wrist supported in a sling, tying a magazine or newspaper, padded wooden splints, or by bandaging the arm to the chest. The lower extremity fractures can be splinted by pillow splint (wrapping an ordinary pillow around the injured limb), padded wooden splints, bandaging both lower limbs together or by inflatable splints, made of double-walled polyvinyl jacket with a zipper fastener. Compound fractures can be splinted the same way but after covering the wound with sterile dressing.

Splintage is removed only at the time of the definitive treatment after radiological evaluation has been done and treatment has been planned. Radiographic evaluation of all multiply injured patients must include a trauma series consisting of:

1. Cervical spine-lateral view (including C_1-C_7 and superior part of T_1)
   Ask for Swimmer's view (Fig. 6.10) if you can't see C_7-T_1
2. Chest-AP view
3. Pelvis-AP view
4. Thoraco lumbar spine-lateral view.

CT scan of head (Fig. 3.5), cervical spine, thorax, abdomen and pelvis with or without contrast may be needed if dictated by the pattern of injury.

SELECTION OF DEFINITIVE TREATMENT

After the radiographic evaluation of the skeletal injury the definitive treatment is selected. Many fractures require no treatment or, just analgesics and restriction of activity with a sling or crutches. Table 3.4 shows common fractures which do not require immobilization in a plaster.

The basic aims of treatment of fracture are:

1. To restore the alignment of the fracture fragments to prevent the deformities in the extremity

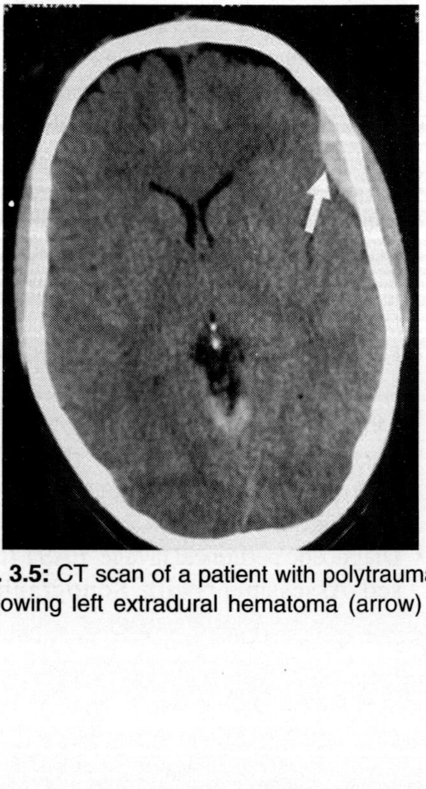

Fig. 3.5: CT scan of a patient with polytrauma showing left extradural hematoma (arrow)

Table 3.4: Common fractures which do not need plaster immobilization/internal fixation

Fracture	*Treatment*
Impacted surgical neck of humerus	Shoulder immobilization
Undisplaced radial head fracture	Sling
Undisplaced olecranon (active extension possible at elbow)	Sling
Distal phalanx of hand/foot	Protect the digit from striking objects/surfaces
Undisplaced greater trochanter	Protected walking with crutches
Undisplaced patella (active extension possible at knee)	Knee immobilizer
Fibula (neck/shaft)	Cane
Undisplaced base of 5th metatarsal	Crepe bandage
Undisplaced calcaneus	Crutches
Stress fractures	Reduce causative activity
Stable/osteoporotic vertebral compression fractures	Brace

2. To secure acceptable apposition of the fracture fragments to facilitate healing
3. To achieve union
4. To restore function so that patient is able to return to his previous occupation, and pursue any physical activity that he desires.

The treatment of fractures, thus, aims to achieve and maintain the reduction (restoration of pre injury position of bony fragments). There are three primary methods to achieve reduction viz. traction, closed reduction and open reduction. Open reduction must always be accompanied by internal fixation to splint the fracture internally. For maintenance of reduction, traction, external immobilization (in the form of plaster, splint or external fixation) or internal fixation can be used. Techniques of traction and plaster application are discussed in Chapter 4. Closed reduction and external immobilization (with plaster/splints/traction) is the treatment of choice whereever possible. The closed reduction of fracture can be done under sedation, regional block or under general anaesthesia (when muscle pull is a major deforming factor). After reduction, suitable external immobilization is performed and the adequacy of reduction checked with radiographs. The joint above and below should be immobilized.

The acceptability of reduction is important because the closed reduction would often not achieve 100% anatomical reduction.

Serial radiographs should be taken at relatively short intervals (5-7 days for 3-4 weeks till the fracture becomes "sticky" and is not likely to redisplace) to ensure that the reduction is maintained. Any loss of position of the fracture fragments during follow up is an indication for remanipulation/open reduction of the fracture.

Function should be preserved in all the joints of the extremity which are not immobilized by active movements and supervised physiotherapy.

Cast Braces: Cast braces are well fitting and are fitted with hinges to allow joint movement. With cast brace, the patient is encouraged to use the limb e.g. patients with cast brace are encouraged to bear full weight on their injured limb much sooner than the conventional splints. However, the cast braces are difficult to apply and require special attention to detail.

Open Reduction and Internal Fixation (ORIF)

The indications for ORIF are:

1. Inability to achieve reduction:
   - Unstable fracture pattern
   - Strong deforming forces (e.g. subtrochanteric fracture of femur)
   - Soft tissue interposition
   - Avulsion fractures with wide separation

- Fractures of the lateral condyle of the humerus where the distal fragment rotates in two planes making the closed reduction of the fracture impossible.

2. Inability to maintain reduction e.g.
   - Unstable fracture pattern-point contact of fracture fragments
   - Fracture of the femoral neck
   - Bulky limb or obese patients making POP immobilization difficult.
3. Loss of reduction after initial acceptable reduction. This often happens when the swelling in the limb comes down and the plaster becomes loose.
4. Nerve or vascular deficit appearing **after** closed reduction of fracture-implying interposition of the neurovascular structures between the fracture fragments e.g. Radial nerve palsy occurring after reduction of the humerus shaft fracture.
5. Intra-articular displaced fractures: To prevent post traumatic osteoarthritis at a later stage.
6. Displaced fracture with disruption of a functionally important mechanism e.g. displaced fracture patella with disruption of extensor mechanism; Displaced fracture olecranon with compromise of active elbow extension due to disruption of triceps attachment.
7. Polytraumatized patient with multiple fractures in different extremities or multiple fractures in the same extremity (e.g. floating knee or floating elbow denoting the occurrence of fracture above as well as below the joint).
8. Fractures in which the blood supply to the limb is jeopardized and the vessels need protection or when the vessels are also injured and need repair.

The commonly used internal fixation devices are Kirschner wires, screws, screws with plates, intramedullary nails-conventional and locked, and various compression/sliding devices for special applications (e.g. Dynamic Hip Screw for intertrochanteric fractures of the femur).

Open reduction has the advantages of allowing a nearly anatomical reduction and allows early discontinuation of external support and restoration of function. However, there are certain disadvantages of internal fixation such as:

1. Loss of fracture hematoma
2. Stripping of the soft tissues to expose and reduce the fracture ends leading to devitalization
   Note: **1 and 2 lead to delayed healing**
3. There is risk of infection. Infection can lead to non union
4. Damage to neurovascular structures may occur during surgery
5. Hardware related problems such as pain at the site of implant, loosening or breakage of implants or refracture after removing the implants.

EXTERNAL FIXATION

External fixation devices have minimal implant-bone contact in the form of pins/wires going through the bone fragments. These pins/wires are captured in a tubular/ring shaped device outside the body to immobilize the bony fragments. External fixation of fracture is indicated in:

1. Compound fractures when the wound is contaminated or there is skin loss because of the risk of infection associated with internal fixation in these cases (Fig. 3.6). External fixators allow the inspection, dressing and reconstruction (skin grafting, etc) of the damaged skin and soft tissues without the risk of loss of reduction of the fracture.

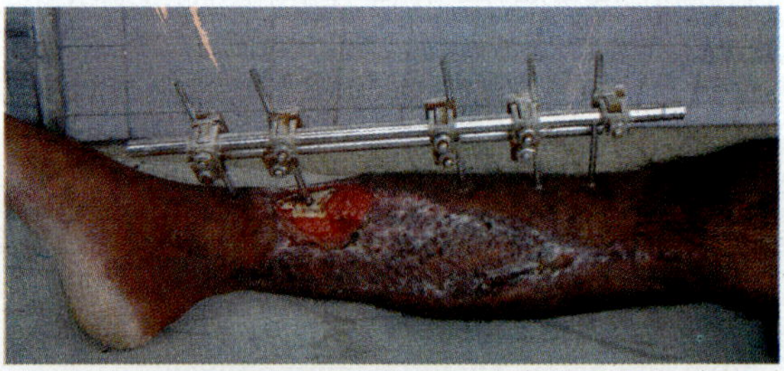

Fig. 3.6: Compound fracture of tibia with loss of overlying soft tissues. External fixator is ideally suited for stabilizing these fractures

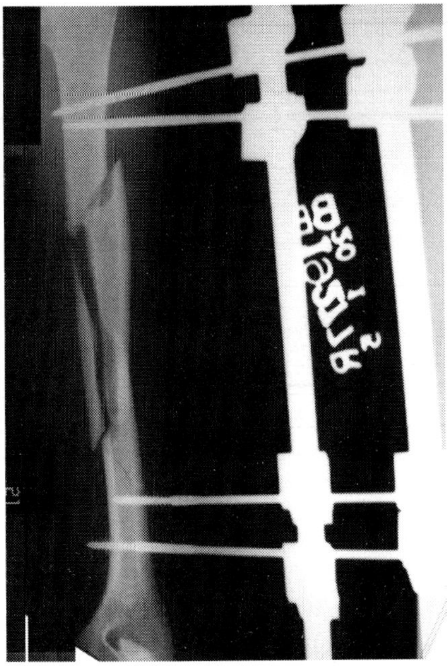

Fig. 3.7: Comminuted fracture of humeral shaft stabilized by external fixator under local anaesthesia in a patient with polytrauma who was unfit for major surgery/anaesthesia

2. In multiply injured patients or elderly patients who are unfit to undergo major operations involving internal fixation of fracture due to major surgical/anaesthetic risk (Fig. 3.7). External fixation can be applied under local anaesthetic in these patients with minimal surgical trauma.
3. As a temporizing/definite treatment method in pelvis fractures (especially the open book type of injury).

The position of bony fragments can be easily adjusted with external fixation.

However, the disadvantages of external fixation are pin-tract infection, delayed union and stiffness of the neighbouring joints due to impalement of the musculotendinous units by the pins.

In general, the following important principles of the management of fractures should be kept in mind:

1. **An open fracture is an emergency.** Early management of open fractures is directed to converting contaminated wounds to clean wounds and further management consists of getting wound cover to convert an open fracture into a closed fracture. An open fracture must be stabilised by external fixation (and rarely, internal fixation if a case presents early-within 6 hours- and has minimal contamination and little disruption/loss of soft tissues) to reduce the risk of infection.
2. Perform a detailed examination to avoid missing a fracture which is not obvious. Table 3.5 depicts the frequently missed fractures.

Table 3.5: Frequently missed fractures

Impacted fracture neck of femur
Fracture of ribs
Skull fractures, especially base of skull
Fracture of odontoid
Fractures of the C7 vertebra
Facial bones, especially around zygoma
Undisplaced fractures of pelvis (especially sacrum)
Fracture of the radial head
Fracture of scaphoid
Fracture dislocations of carpus, especially Lunate
Fractures of talus
Fracture dislocations of tarso-metatarsal joints
Stress/fatigue fractures

An X-ray of pelvis must be taken in all patients with any major lower limb trauma to rule out pelvic/hip injuries (Fig. 3.8).

3. Head/abdominal/chest trauma take precedence over skeletal trauma except in case of treatment of dislocation of hip which takes precedence over other injuries.
4. Cervical spine X-rays must be taken in all patients with head injury/unconscious state/inebriated state due to alcohol etc. to rule out cervical spine injury.

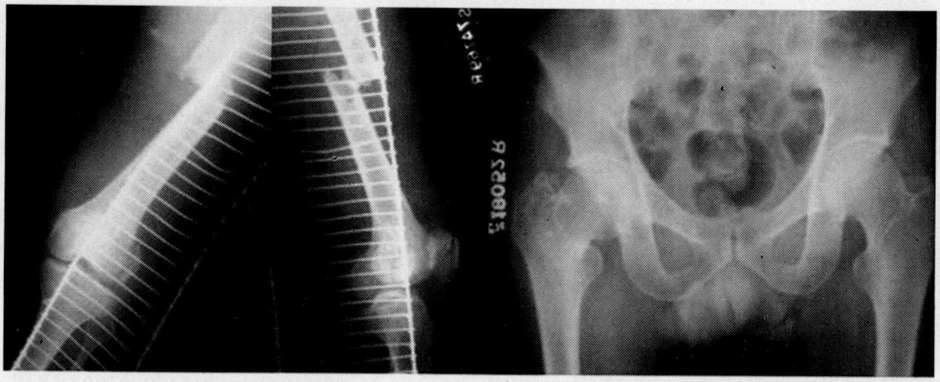

Fig. 3.8: AP (left) and lateral (middle) X-rays of patient with femoral shaft fracture. This patient also had fracture of femoral neck (right). These fractures are often missed. Also note comminuted fracture patella and fracture of the lateral femoral condyle.

5. Intravenous access must be established in all patients with any pelvis/femur and/or multiple long bone fractures.
6. All fractures must be splinted immediately to relieve pain and prevent damage to soft tissues.
7. Always obtain appropriate radiographs:
   a. At least in two planes at right angles to each other.
   b. Include a joint above and a joint below the area of injury in the X-rays.
   c. Obtain oblique/special views whenever necessary.
   d. Opposite extremity radiographs whenever a questionable fracture is present, especially in children.
8. Intra-articular fractures at all ages and epiphyseal injuries in children must be reduced anatomically to prevent late onset of osteoarthritis or growth disturbances respectively.
9. Whenever one bone of forearm or leg is fractured and becomes shortened or angulated, it cannot do so without breaking the other bone or dislocating the proximal or the distal joint between the two bones.
10. Avulsion fracture near a joint may compromise the function of a ligament and/or tendon and should be evaluated carefully for instability.
11. Irreducibility of fracture may signify soft tissue interposition between the fracture ends.
12. Fractures associated with significant soft tissue injury and swelling and fractures around elbow are preferably treated in a slab to accommodate swelling in the limb.
13. **ALWAYS** assess the distal neurovascular status and movement of digits before treatment and after the treatment.
14. Multiple fractures in the same extremity and/or fractures in bilateral limbs should be operated and internally fixed early.
15. The fractures and dislocations in the upper limb take 6 weeks and 3 weeks respectively to heal in adults. The figures are approximatley 12 weeks and 6 weeks respectively for fractures and dislocations in the lower limbs.

PRINCIPLES OF TREATMENT OF FRACTURES IN CHILDREN

The fractures in children differ from the adults in several respects. The bones in children are more porous and resilient and often tolerate greater angulation/deformation before fracture. Epiphysis at the end of bone is a weak point and often fails resulting in epiphyseal injuries. Dislocations, except of the patellofemoral joint, are rare as the ligaments are strong. Children suffer fractures in elbow region and clavicle more commonly while the fractures of femoral neck, spinal injuries, intra-articular fractures and fractures of the carpal bones are rarely seen in children. Fracture heal quickly and predictably and non union is rare because of active periosteum and abundant blood supply to the bone. Fractures are less complicated and are almost always treated with closed methods, with a few exceptions. Physiotherapy after the fracture has healed is usually unnecessary. Continued growth of the bone in children after the bone has healed will allow for some correction and realignment of minor deformities.

REMODELLING OF DEFORMITIES IN CHILDREN

1. Mild angular deformities frequently correct with growth and the amount of correction depends on the amount and direction of angulation, age of the child, and distance of the fracture from the end of bone.
   - Correction is more complete with milder deformities.
   - Correction is also more complete if the angulation is in the same plane of motion as the nearest joint. Deformities in other planes will persist.
   - Younger the age, better the remodelling of deformities.
   - Farther the deformity from the end of the bone, lesser the remodeling i.e. deformities closer to joints remodel faster.
2. Rotational deformities do not correct with growth.
3. Overlapping of bones often leads to acceleration of growth in children and tibia and femur may overgrow upto one centimeter following a displaced fracture. Therefore, slight overlapping of bone fragments is occasionally desirable in tibia/femur fracture in children as the correction of this overriding may lead to lengthening of the injured limb subsequently with growth.

EPIPHYSEAL INJURIES

Epiphyseal injuries typically occur in the growing skeleton. The injuries occur through the weakest

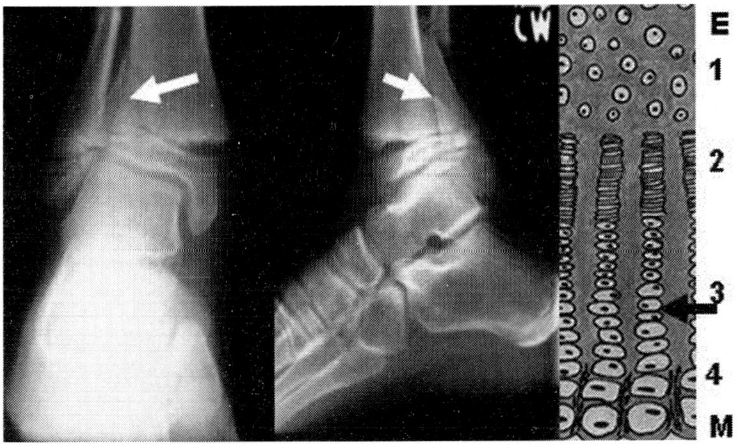

Fig. 3.9: Type II epiphyseal injury of distal tibial epiphysis. Note the Thurston Holland sign (White arrows) on the AP and lateral X-rays. These injuries occur through the zone of hypertrophy (Zone 3—black arrow) (E: Epiphyseal or articular end, 1: Zone of resting cartilage, 2: Zone of proliferating cartilage, 3: Zone of hypertrophy, 4: Zone of provisional calcification, M: Metaphyseal end of growth plate)

zone of the epiphyseal (or growth) plate i.e. the zone of hypertrophic cartilage. These injuries are classified by Salter-Harris classification. Type I and II are transverse fractures across the growth plate and heal normally. Type II epiphyseal injuries are the most common and invariably have a triangular metaphyseal fragment (Thurston Holland Sign) (Fig. 3.9). The most common epiphyseal injury in children occurs at the distal radial epiphysis. Growth disturbances do not occur. In type III and IV injuries, the fracture traverses the growth plate vertically and growth disturbances occur frequently. These injuries are frequently intra-articular and need accurate reduction by surgical method to restore the joint surface. Cross-union or bony block may form across the epiphyseal plate and lead to angular deformity with growth.

Type V epiphyseal injuries result from crushing of the epiphyseal plate and have the worst prognosis.

Caution: Epiphyseal injuries may often be missed or an epiphyseal plate may be mistaken as fracture. For all such doubtful cases in children, X- rays of the opposite extremity must be taken for comparison.

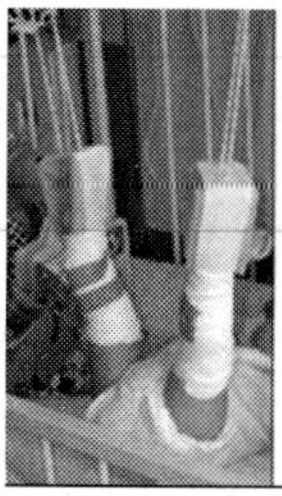

4 Conservative Treatment of Fractures

Traction, Casting, Slings, Splints

Reduction and immobilization of the bones ensures (a) union without deformity, and (b) prevention of pain at the fracture site.

A fracture may be immobilized by traction, splint, sling and cast, or operatively by external or internal fixation.

TRACTION

Implies application of force along the long axis of a bone or the axial skeleton. Immediately following a fracture, the muscles around the broken bone go into spasm and cause deformity and shortening of the limb as they act as a bowstring. [The same (bow string) effect causes the loss of position of fractures]. Pulling on the limb with injury (Traction) draws the fragments in line, maintains the reduction i.e. prevents deformity and shortening, overcomes muscle power and relieves pain by limiting movements at the fracture site. Continuous traction can be applied either to the skin or the bony skeleton.

Skin Traction

A soft dressing is bound to limbs and a traction apparatus is attached to the soft dressing (Fig. 4.1). Felt pads are used to protect bony prominences. The weight is applied to the bone indirectly via the soft tissues. The upper limit of weight which can be used with skin traction is 5 kg (12 pounds) as too much weight can disrupt the skin and soft tissues. Therefore, skin traction is suitable only in children and as a temporary measure in adults. Elderly patients, patients with rheumatoid arthritis, patients on steroids, diabetics and patients with poor peripheral circulation are prone to soft tissue/ skin complications and skin traction should be avoided in these patients.

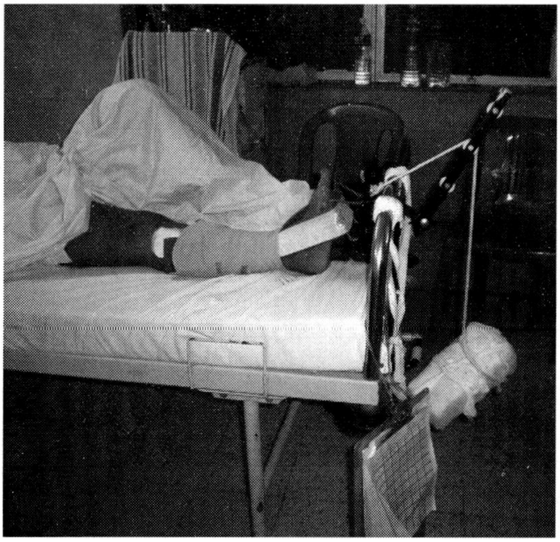

Fig. 4.1: Skin traction

Complications of Skin Traction

1. *Skin damage:* Allergic dermatitis, blister formation and/or peeling of skin may occur. Peripheral edema is common when the bandages are too tight or slip.
2. *Circulatory impairment:* If bandages are applied too tightly, circulatory impairment may occur especially in patients with swelling, atherosclerosis or diabetes.

3. *Pressure areas:* Especially over bony prominences.
4. *Compression of nerve:* Especially the common peroneal nerve at fibular neck if skin traction extends proximally to the fibular neck and bandages are applied tightly.
5. *Compartment syndrome* may occur the bandage is applied tightly. It is a particularly serious complication (also see page 41-42)
6. *Stiffness of the joints* may occur due to immobilisation.

Skeletal Traction

The traction is applied to the pins passed through the bone. Either smooth pins with trocar point (Steinmann pin) or threaded pins (Denham pin) can be used (Fig. 4.2). The threads of Denham pins grip the bone and prevent lateral slippage. A Bohler stirrup holds the pin and provides attachment to the traction cord and weights.

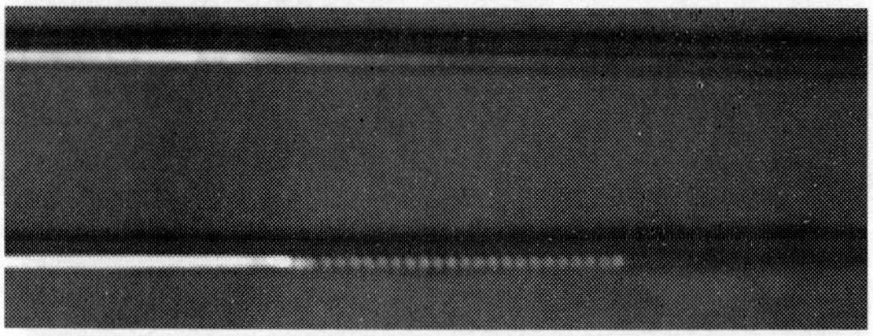

Fig. 4.2: Pins used for skeletal traction (Top) Smooth (Steinmann) pin; (Bottom) Threaded (Denham) pin.

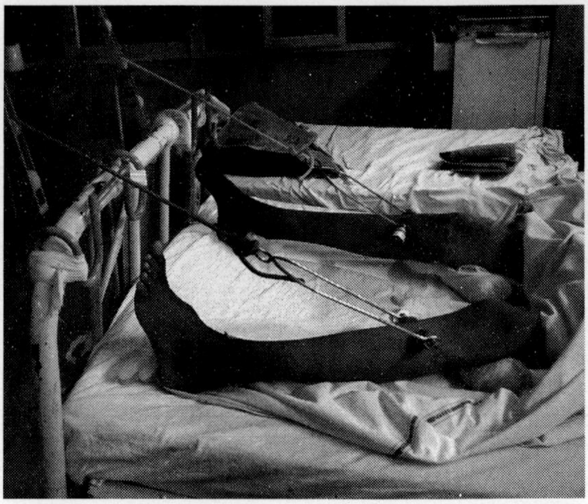

Fig. 4.3: Bilateral upper tibial pin skeletal traction through Steinmann pins using Bohler's stirrups

The most common sites of insertion of skeletal pins are:

- Upper tibia (Fig. 4.3)
- Calcaneum
- Lower femur (supracondylar)
- Lower tibia (supra malleolar)
- Skull

Olecranon pin traction and skeletal traction in children is applied using a Kirschner wire (K-wire) tensioned using a special device (K-wire tensioner). Key precautions to be taken while applying skeletal traction are shown in Table 4.1.

Table 4.1: Key precautions while setting up skeletal traction

Step	*Explanation*
1. Introduce the pin from the side of an important neurovascular structure e.g. lateral side for upper tibial pin to prevent injury to common peroneal nerve	It is easier to avoid impaling the key structure this way. You may not have adequate control on where the pin may come out of bone on opposite side.
2. When using local anesthesia infiltrate the skin and periosteum carefully at points of entry and exit	Periosteum has pain sensations and must be infiltrated.
3. Drill the pin through the bone with a hand drill or T handle	Power drill may cause necrosis of bone by generating heat—Ring sequetrum may form. Hammering may cause fracture
4. A threaded pin (Denham) is better than Steinmann pin	Threads prevent loosening. But exercise care while removing Denham pin–unscrew; do not pull
5. Keep the point of entry clean. Do not wind bandage around the pin like a cleat	To avoid skin necrosis and pin tract infection.
6. Cap the sharp end of traction pin with penicillin vial or plastic	Capping avoids injury by pointed tip of traction pin

If the Bohler stirrup digs on the lower limb, or the skeletal traction is unable to control the rotation of the limb, two traction ropes with two pullies, wide apart and attached to the two ends of the traction pin should be used.

Complications of skeletal traction:

1. Injury of neurovascular structures (if proper attention is not paid to details).
2. Pin tract infection and loosening of pin, ring sequestrum.
3. Over distraction.
4. Loss of position.
5. Pressure sores.

Some Special Traction Methods

Gallows Traction (Bryant's method)

Used for treating a child below 2 years of age with a fracture of the femoral shaft. It is a fixed skin traction method which suspends the patients up by the injured limb and leaves them hanging till healing has occurred (Fig. 4.4). This traction should not be used in older or heavier children as nerve compression and ischemia of the distal leg and foot can occur especially if the knee hyperextends.

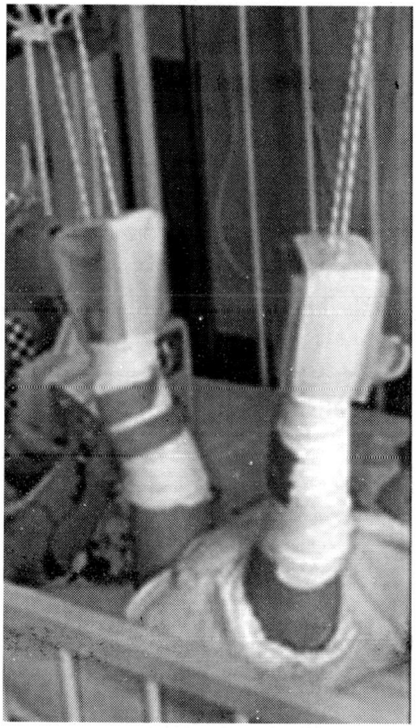

Fig. 4.4: Gallow's traction

Perkin's Traction

Simple sliding skeletal traction over a pillow. Used in adults with femoral shaft fracture.

Fixed Traction with Splint

Used for transporting patients with femoral shaft fracture or as initial temporizing measure. A Spanish windlass is used to tighten the traction cords and increase the pull of traction.

Hamilton Russel Traction

Used for trochanteric fracture; can be applied using skin or skeletal traction. The traction uses a single cord to apply a horizontal force which is twice the vertical force by using a three-pully system for the horizontal run of the cord.

90-90 Traction (Fig 4.5)

Traction of 90-90 type is used for treating femoral shaft fractures when there is wound on the posterior aspect of thigh. Presence of significant soft tissue and skin loss, however, is better managed by external fixation these days.

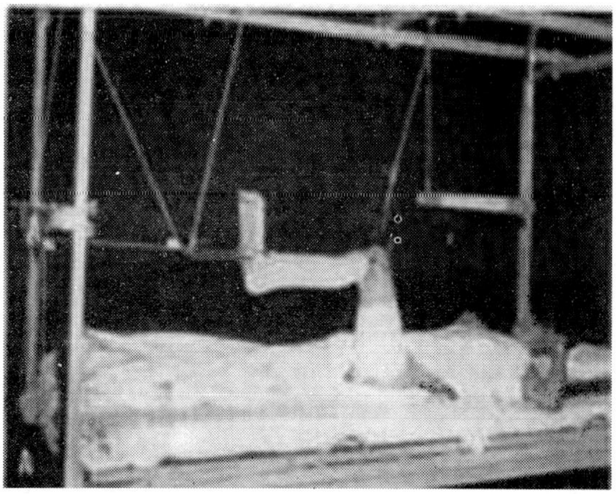

Fig. 4.5: 90-90 traction

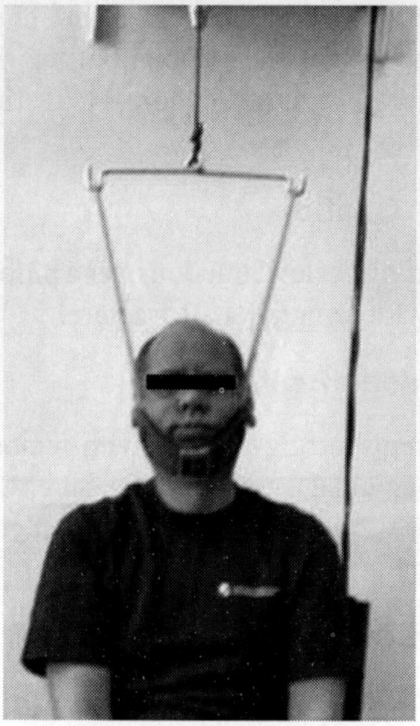

Fig. 4.6: Head Halter traction

Skull Traction

Skull traction is used for the cervical spine injuries to prevent further damage to the spinal cord, provide stability while healing of fracture or dislocation occurs and allow nursing by moving the patient to prevent bed sores and pneumonia.

Skull traction can be applied by Halter traction as a temporary measure (Fig. 4.6) or by skull tongs. Crutchfield tongs are inserted into the outer table of the skull under local anaesthetic (Fig. 4.7). Skull traction can be used to reduce facet joint dislocation by steady traction without anaesthesia rather than risking a manipulation under a general anaesthesia. A rule of thumb is to use 4.5 kg (10 lb) weight in traction to overcome the weight of head and 2.25 kg (5 lb) for every inter space. The means that traction is with 6.75 kg (15 lb) initially and increased by 2.25 kg (5 lb) every 15-30 minutes upto 15.75-18 kg (35-40 lb) with periodic X-rays to check whether the reduction has occurred or not.

Halo traction ring allows traction through a plaster or PVC jacket and allows the patient to be ambulant, prevents bed sores and allows easier multi-directional control of the traction (Fig. 4.8).

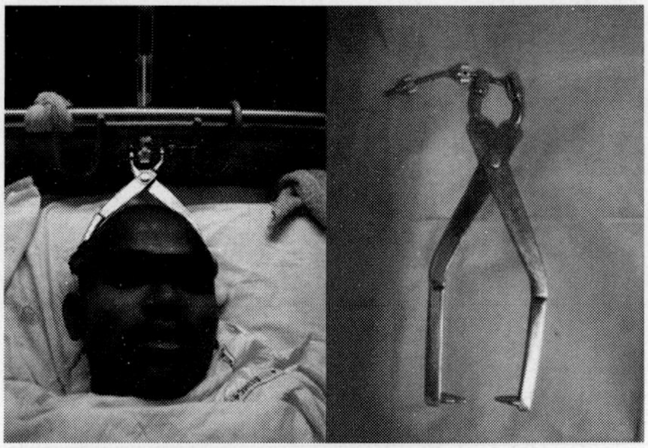

Fig. 4.7: (Left) Skull traction using Crutchfield tongs (Right) Crutchfield tongs

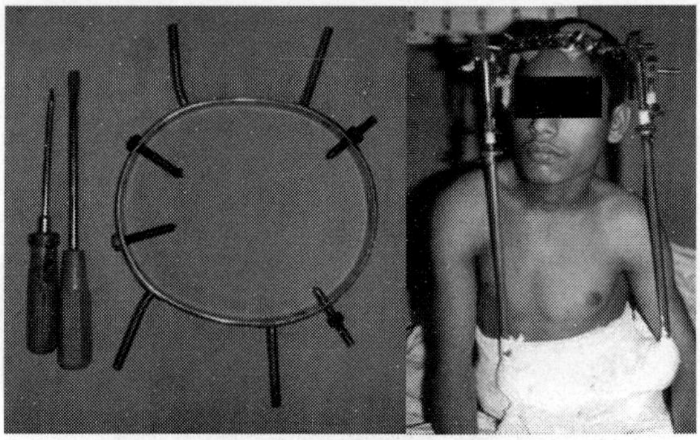

Fig. 4.8: (Left) Halo ring (Right); Halopelvic traction using plaster jacket

Dunlop Traction

Dunlop Traction is used for the supracondylar fractures of the humerus. It entails longitudinal skin traction along the long axis of the forearm with elbow flexed 90 degrees and a second weight applied vertically through a sling on the lower part of the arm to counter the tendency for anterior angulation.

CASTING

Casts are devices which hold a fracture steady by setting hard around the limb. Casting is the mainstay of treatment for most fractures. Casts reduce pain and keep an undisplaced or recently manipulated fracture in position until adequate healing occurs.

The plaster can be applied as:

1. Unpadded plater: a 'skin-tight' plaster which fits snugly over the limb. However this types of plaster has to be applied carefully as it can cause sores if there are any indentations in the plaster. Also, it does not accommodate any swelling and can cause circulatory embarrassment.
2. Padded plaster is applied around abundant padding and is safer. This is the most popular technique.

Casting Materials

Casting bandages consist of bandages impregnated with casting material. Plaster of Paris and fiberglass are the primary casting materials.

Plaster of Paris (POP) is the best known casting material. It is a high quality gypsum which originally came from Montmartre. It is cheap, light, comparatively soft, porous (skin can breathe), easy to apply, safe, fairly easy to remove, is non allergenic, and has a long shelf life. Its main disadvantages are that it disintegrates when wet and is hard enough to take patient's weight only after 2-3 days. Plaster of Paris bandages consists of a tough open weave fabric coated with hemihydrated calcium sulphate powder ($CaSO_4$ ½ H_2O). When dipped in water the plaster becomes the hard and crystalline hydrated calcium sulphate. The chemical reaction is exothermic and the plater becomes warm as it sets.

$$(CaSO_4)_2\,H_2O + 3H_2O \rightarrow 2\,(CaSO_4.\,2H_2O) + \text{Heat}$$

Plaster of Paris is preferred by most orthopaedic surgeons. Modern materials, such as resins and fiberglass have not displaced plaster of paris.

Fiberglass is light weight, water resistent, durable and neat. In addition, it is radiolucent and allows early weight bearing. However, it is expensive, hard to apply, non porous and often needs a special diamond edged power saw to remove the casts.

Applying a Plaster

Applying a good plaster needs a lot of practice. The key points which must be kept in mind while apply the cast include:

1. Use appropriate (3-4 layers) soft wool or cotton padding especially over the bony areas to avoid pressure sores, preferably over a thin layer of stockinette so that the padding will not roll inside the cast and cause uncomfortable ridges.
   Caution: Too much padding near the fracture site can led to inadequate immobilization.
2. *Check water temperature:* Warmer the water, shorter the curing time of casting material. Beginners can use cold water as it gives more time to apply the cast.
3. *Dipping:* Dip the cast bandage **after** identifying the edge and unroll it for a couple of inches (to avoid difficulty in finding the edge after wetting). Hold the bandage lightly so that water can penetrate to the centre of the bandage. Hold it under the water till the bubbles stop, then drain it till the drips stop. Do not wring it out.
4. *Application:* Roll the bandage gently and carefully around the limb. Do not pull the bandage tight. Tuck the edges when there is change in the girth of the limb. Gently mould the cast so that it conforms to the shape of limb. In most cases the joint above and below must be immobilized and cast must be reinforced by bridging across the joint(s). The joints must be immobilised in the position of function. The wrist and hand, for example, are immobilized in the grasping position; the elbow in 90° flexion, ankle in neutral position, forearm usually in mid prone position and knee usually in 20-30° of flexion. However, for the treatment of some fractures these principles have to be violated to optimize the outcome.
5. *Avoid:*
   a. Applying the cast on limb with encircling bandages, rings, bangles etc.
   b. Applying the cast too lightly.

c. Excessive molding
d. Creating indentations in the cast.
e. Hard wrinkles in the cast. This is especially common around the joints. A trick to avoid hard wrinkles in the cast is to flex the joint to 100° degrees if it has to be immobilized in 90° flexion, apply the cast and then place the limb in the correct position. This trick prevents pressure sores at the flexure crease.

6. *Check after the plaster has been applied:*
   a. Tips of the digits: Should never be hidden by the plaster.
   b. Rotation of the limb: especially in fractures of tibial shaft which can easily rotate out of true anatomical alignment.
   c. Edges: Should not be sharp/should not dig in the skin; evert or bend the edges if sharp edges are present.
   d. Circulation: Capillary refill, color, sensation and the movements should be normal. Ensure that the plaster is not too tight and is not going to prevent venous return leading to venous tourniquet effect.
   e. Integrity of cast: Check for crack which might have appeared if limb is moved during application, weak areas, indentations, creases
   f. X-rays: If manipulation was done to reduce the bony fragments. Patient should be advised about the need for **weekly** check X-ray to check alignment of fracture fragments for the next 3-4 weeks till the fracture becomes "sticky". This is because the fragments may redisplace in plaster especially when the swelling comes down.

7. *Advise:*
   a. Danger signs: Advise to return immediately if there is increased numbness, excessive swelling, bluish discoloration of digits, sensation of cast being too tight, constant irritation or severe pain. **Provide Written instructions.**
   b. Limb elevation, especially for the first 3-5 days.
   c. Digit movements and movements of all the joints of the extremity which are not immobilised e.g. shoulder movement must be performed regularly after Colles' fracture to avoid stiffness.
   d. Ambulation: especially in lower extremity injuries. The patient should be advised whether he should walk non weight bearing, partial weight bearing or full weight bearing. Advise plaster boot, slipper or walking heel to assist walking with a cast when allowed.
   e. Care of the plaster to avoid wetting the cast (especially for spicas and in young children) or report if the cast is damaged and/or allows movements which it was preventing earlier.
   f. The next follow up including the need for next X-ray. Normally all patients should be checked again within 24 hours of application (including weekends).
   g. Expected duration for which the cast will be kept.

POP Slab or Splint is used when considerable swelling in the limb is expected in which case casts can be potentially dangerous. The slab is especially useful for elbow injuries in children and in soft tissue injuries. The limb is wrapped in cast padding and 10 to 12 thicknesses of plaster of the appropriate length are dipped in water, taken out, fitted to the extremity and held in place with loose cotton bandages. The joints should be immobilised in the "position of function". Slabs are not very strong and when applied on lower extremity, do not allow weight bearing.

Pins and Plaster

A plaster just holds a limb to its length and does not prevent shortening. Some oblique and/or comminuted fractures can result in shortening, the bone ends sliding upon one another. This is commonly seen in tibial shaft fractures. If a pin is passed through calcaneus or the distal fragment and incorporated in the plaster, this tendency is

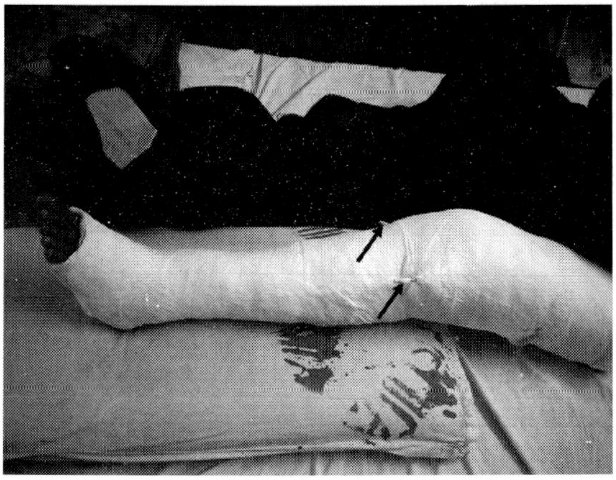

Fig. 4.9: Pins and plaster pins (arrows) passed through the bone are incorporated in plaster to maintain reduction

counteracted (Fig. 4.9). This pin can be removed once the fracture is sticky.

Note: The availability of the external fixator and closed nailing techniques have reduced the need for this technique.

Window, Splitting, Bivalving, Wedging or Removing Casts

Basic equipment for these techniques includes a large and a small pair of plaster shears, a pair of bandage scissors and a pair of plaster spreaders. In addition, an oscillating saw should be available.

Window: The situation of wounds or other soft tissue problems should be marked immediately upon the plaster so that a window may be cut in the plaster to permit monitoring of wound and dressing.

Splitting: The plaster must be split when the swelling occurs or is expected in the limb. The split must be along the entire length and through the entire thickness of both the cast and the fabric, down to the skin. This can be easily accomplished with the oscillating saw and bandage scissors.

Bivalving the cast means diving it along its whole length at two opposite locations (on each side) so that the plaster is cut into two halves and one half of the plaster shell can be lifted off. Bivalved segments of the cast are also often used as night splints to prevent the deformities or maintain the correction of deformities.

Removal of plaster is indicated when the:

a. Fracture is clinically united i.e. there is no local pain, tenderness, or movement at the fracture site.
b. Fracture is radiologically united (see Chapter 2) [For this, the X-ray should be taken out of plaster] and,
c. There is no significant risks of re fracture providing the patient abides by instructions.

Removal is easy when the plater is bivalved. The patient should be warned that the limb will be stiff for some time and regular physiotherapy and use of the limb will be required to restore function.

Wedging: is an excellent technique which allows the surgeon to realign a fracture which was either inadquately reduced or has slipped. The plaster is circumferentially split for 50-75 percent of its surface at the site corresponding to the fracture. The plaster edges are then spread apart (Open wedge technique) and the little pieces of wood, cut to a length judged adequate to correct the alignment are inserted to maintain the gap created. The plaster is then reconstituted with plaster bandages and the position of fracture fragment confirmed on the X-rays (Fig. 4.10).

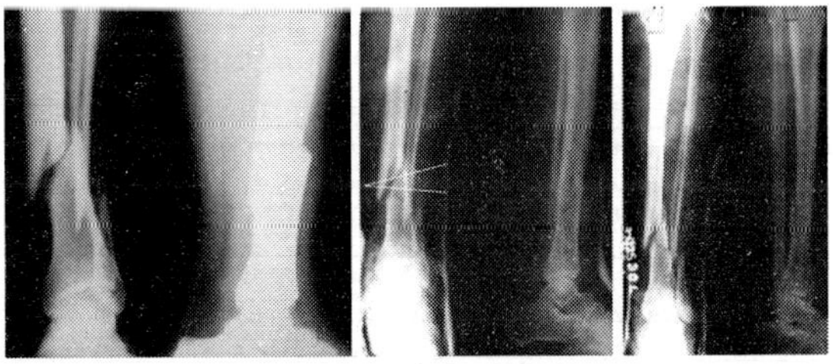

Fig. 4.10: Wedging of cast. (Extreme left) Fracture both bones of leg (Middle) Position following manipulation and plaster application shows medial angulation. An open wedge (shown by lines) in the plaster on the lateral side improved the reduction (Right)

Complications of Plaster Cast Treatment

1. Circulatory embarrassment, soft tissue problems.
2. Compartment syndrome
3. Pressure sores, skin chafing, plaster blisters, undiagnosed wound infection.
4. Joint stiffness due to immobilisation leading to adverse changes in articular cartilage.
5. Wasting of muscles, weakness, atrophy of skin, and stiffness of joints are grouped together and called "Fracture Disease" which is common after plaster immobilization.
6. Disuse osteoporosis of bones.
7. Malunion where plaster is unable to maintain alignment of fragments.
8. Non union when bone ends which become too mobile in plaster proceed to non union.

EMERGENCY SPLINTS

Definition: Splint is an orthopaedic device for immobilization, restraint or support of any part of the body. Knowledge of these is necessary for an early and effective trauma care management.

Objectives: In trauma care they are used-

- To maintain the alignment of the extremity
- To provide stability at the fracture site by providing immobilization
- To enforce specific directional control
- To provide attachment for devices and traction.

Splints also play an important role in the management of other orthopaedic conditions like infection, nerve injuries, congenital disorders, neuromuscular disorders etc.

Terminology: Various terms are used for splints:

1. *Make–do splints:* They are temporary splints made from commonly available materials. One can use an umbrella, folded newspaper, pillow, rigid cardboard, wooden sticks etc. for temporary splinting of extremities. They are especially useful for emergency transportation to a place for definitive management.

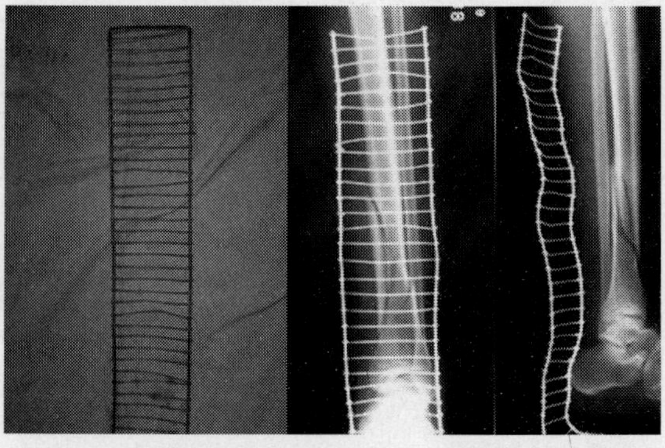

Fig. 4.11: Cramer wire splint. This splint is extremely useful for emergency splintage of extremity fractures

2. *Commercial splints:* These splints are commercially available. They can be:
   - Temporary e.g. Cramer-wire splint (Fig 4.11).
   - Definitive e.g. Conservative management of fracture shaft of femur in a Thomas splint (Fig. 4.12).
3. They can be named according to anatomical location and extent e.g. Upper extremity splints, lower extremity splints, distal, proximal, shoulder, thumb spica splint etc.
4. *Air splints:* This splint is wrapped around the extremity and closed by its zipper and then inflated by flowing air into the mouth tube. They should not be used for extended periods.

Examples of Common Emergency Splints

- *Emergency splinting of spine:* All patients with suspected or diagnosed spinal injuries should be immobilized with a backboard. Sandbags, pillows, rolled towels can be put on either side of cervical spine to immobilize it. Various commercially available neck collars in different sizes can be used for this purpose (Fig. 4.13). Philadelphia collars also have opening for tracheostomy (Fig. 4.14). A temporary collar of desired size and width can be made by filling cotton inside stockinet; it is especially useful in children.

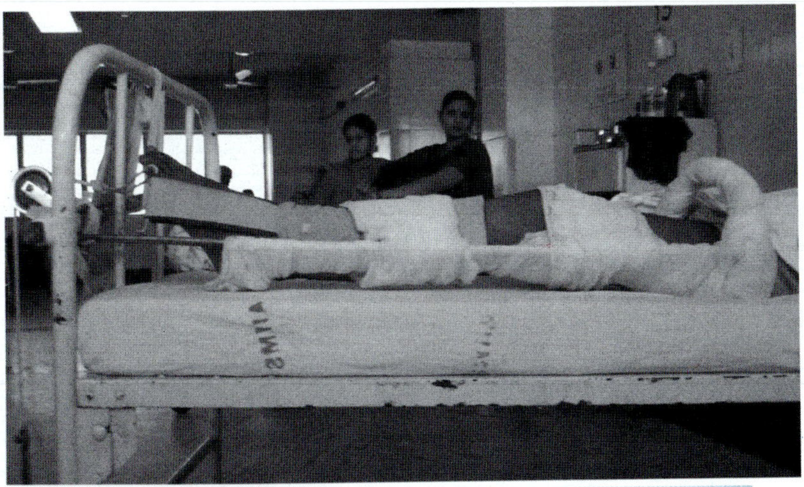

Fig. 4.12: Thomas splint. This splint can be used for conservative treatment of femoral shaft fractures

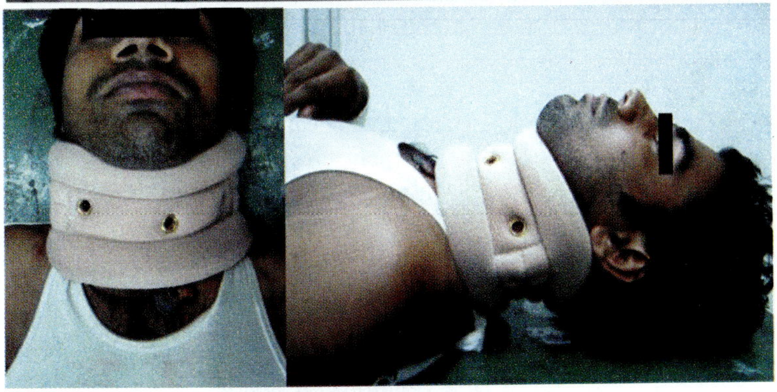

Fig. 4.13: (Soft) Cervical collar. This is an extremely useful splint for immobilization of cervical spine

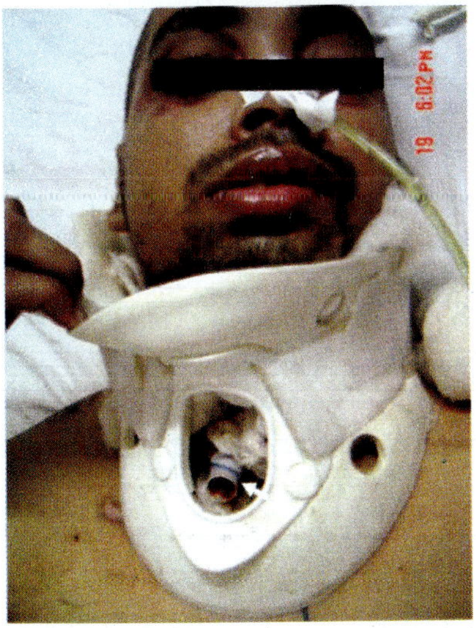

Fig. 4.14: (Hard) Philadelphia collar. Note that it has an opening in front to accommodate tracheostomy tube (arrow)

- *Upper extremity splinting:* Various examples are:
  1. Figure of '8' splint: used for clavicular fractures.
  2. Velpeau and sling and swathe bandages: Used for shoulder dislocations, proximal humeral fractures.
  3. Cock up splint for Radial nerve palsy as following humeral shaft fracture (Fig 4.15).
  4. Mallet finger splint, thumb spica splint etc.
- *Lower extremity splinting*: Various examples are:
  - *Thomas splint (Fig 4.12):* This commonly used splint was devised by Hugh Owen Thomas. It is used for femoral shaft fractures and occasionally for knee injuries. It has got a ring and two sides bar joined distally. Ideal size of ring is 2 inches greater than circumference of proximal thigh. The

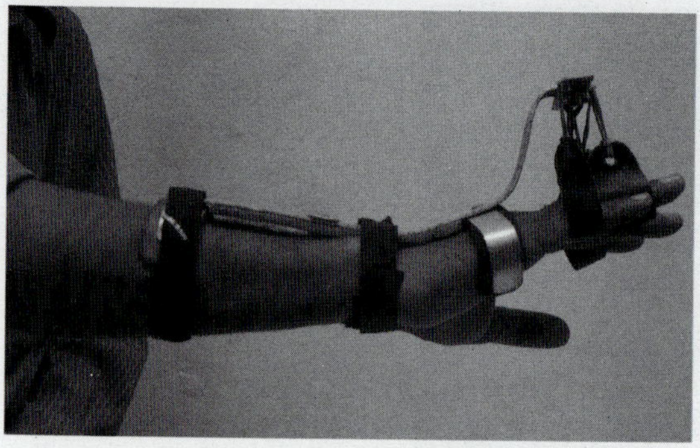

Fig. 4.15: Cock up splint

ring is attached to inside bar at an angle of 120 degrees. It engages the ischial tuberosity for counter traction. The outside bar is curved proximally to accommodate the greater trochanter. The length of Thomas splint is measured by adding 6 inches into the length from medial side of groin to the heel.

– *Bohler-Braun splint (Fig 4.16):* This is another commonly used splint for lower extremity. It has got advantage over Thomas splint as it has no ring. The parts of the splint are:
  - Horizontal elevated part: to support the leg on slings
  - Inclined part: to support the thigh on slings
  - Pulleys: over which the rope passes, and to which weights are attached.

  Disadvantages include:
  - The splint is merely a cradle for the limb.
  - The position of the pulleys cannot be altered.
  - Size of the splint often does not fit the limb as exactly as might be desired.

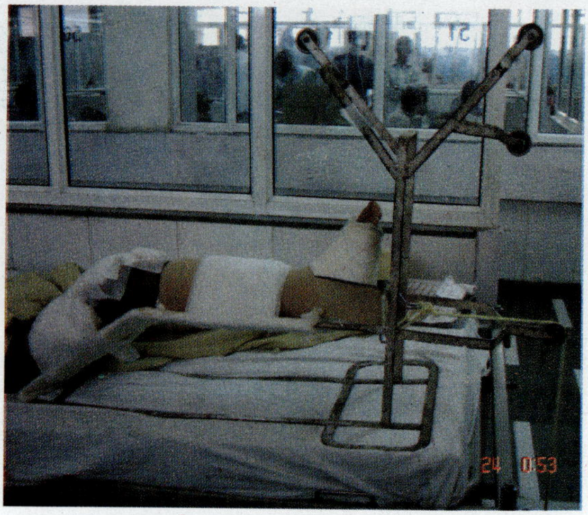

Fig. 4.16: Bohler Braun splint

  - Lateral bowing at the fracture site is common because the splint and the distal fragment are fixed to the frame while the patient and the proximal fragment can move sideways leaving the frame behind!
  - Nursing care is difficult because the patient is not as mobile as he would be, for example, in a Thomas's splint.

Care of a patient in a splint:

a. Avoid circulatory embarrassment by applying splint in such a way as to prevent pressure over bony prominences and tourniquet effect.
b. For closed fractures, alignment should be restored before applying splint.
c. For compound fractures, wound should be covered by moist saline dressing with aseptic technique and alignment should be restored.
d. Any neurovascular compromise should be detected early and managed accordingly.
e. Daily checking and adjustments are must.

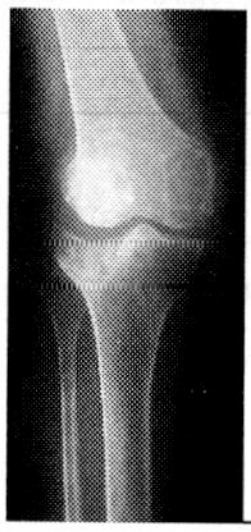

5

Complications of Fractures

Immediate, Early or Intermediate, Late, Complications affecting joints, Fracture emergencies

Fractures are prone to a number of complications, some of them serious. These complications may arise at the time of the initial injury or during the subsequent management of these injuries. The complications of fracture may be (a) General (systemic) complications, (b) Local viz. those involving other structures in the area of fracture (such as neurovascular structures, other soft tissues, joints in the vicinity of injured bone), or, (c) particular to fracture as a whole. The complications may be osseous tissue complications (delayed union, non union, osteomyelitis) or soft tissue complications (neurovascular injuries, compartment syndrome etc). However, conventionally or more commonly, the complications of fractures are classified according to the time after injury when they occur. So they can be immediate, early or intermediate and late complications.

IMMEDIATE COMPLICATIONS (Table 5.1)

Occur at the time of injury. Some of these complications are life threatening and require urgent action. Life threatening conditions which may occur with the fractures include hemorrhage, head injury, fat embolism and pulmonary embolism.

Table 5.1: Immediate complications of fractures

- Hemorrhage
- Injury to important internal organs
- Injury to arteries
- Injury to nerves
- Skin loss or damage

Other life threatening conditions associated with fractures are gas gangrene and tetanus though they occur after a few days.

1. **Severe hemorrhage** is the most common life threatening condition associated with fractures. Bleeding, internal (especially pelvis or femur fractures) or external (compound fractures) leads to hypovolaemic shock. There is decreased blood flow and oxygenation to the tissues. It should be remembered that the circulating blood volume is 7% of body weight in adult and 8-9 % body weight in children. The fall in systolic blood pressure may be compensated well and blood pressure may be maintained with loss upto 30% of blood volume. There are 4 classes of haemorrhage: Class I (upto 15% blood loss), II (15-30% loss), III (30-40% loss) and IV (> 40% loss of circulating blood volume). Class I and II are treated with crystalloid infusions, class III need crystalloids and blood replacement while class IV is a critical condition and aggressive measures have to be taken to save the life of the patient.
2. **Injury to important internal organs** (brain, lung, liver etc.). Skull fractures may lead to injury to the brain. A fractured rib may puncture lung and cause pneumothorax. Broken ribs can also cause laceration of the liver. A pelvis fracture can damage urethra, bladder or bowel. A fractured sternum can lead to rupture of aorta and death due to exsanguination. Fractures of the face or mandible can lead to asphyxia due to obstructed airway.

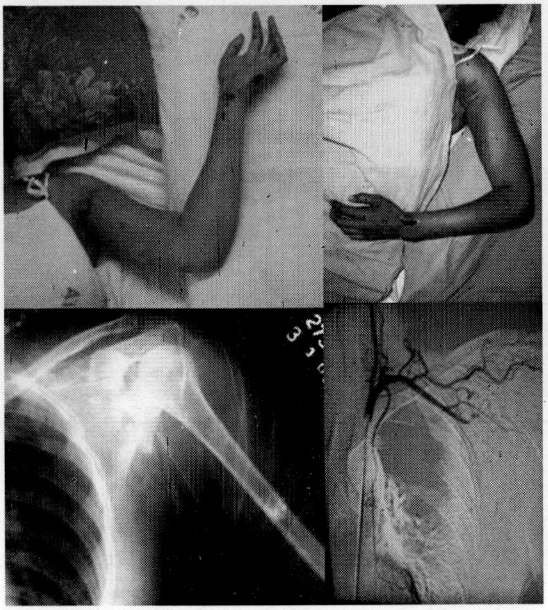

Fig. 5.1: This 40-year-old lady (a victim of RTA) presented with signs of gangrene (Top). X-rays showed scapular fracture (bottom left) and angiography revealed axillary artery injury (Bottom right)

3. **Injury to local vessels (Fig. 5.1).** Vascular injaries occur in a small percentage of fractures. Arterial injuries are most common with dislocations, fractures with penetrating injuries, gunshot wounds or at certain particular sites (e.g. around elbow in supra condylar humerus fracture, around knee after dislocation, following shoulder dislocation, injury to aorta in fractures of 4th and 5th thoracic vertebrae and, middle meningeal artery in temporoparietal skull fractures). There may be damage to the vessel itself which can be open injury (Partial or complete tear, A-V fistula) or a lesion in continuity (stretching or angulation of vessel over the fracture fragment, spasm, intimal tear).

The vascular injury may become apparent immediately when due to disruption of the vessel, acute torsion or kinking of the vessel by fracture fragment or the position of the extremity. One should remember, however, that the vascular injury may become apparent after 24-72 hours and this is particularly common after the knee dislocations. One must always have a high index of suspicion for vascular injuries and one must be aware of the triad of pain, pallor and pulselessness as these are the cardinal signs of arterial insufficiency.

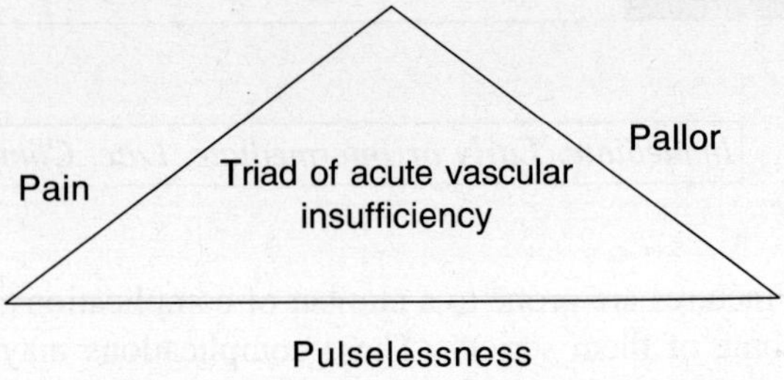

The adverse outcomes of arterial injuries can be minimized by following the steps mentioned below.

a. Distal circulation must be assessed in **all** patients with a fracture or dislocation. Apart from the triad, look for capillary refill (slow refill taking > 3 seconds suggests vascular injury), temperature and digit movements.
b. When dislocations or displaced fractures are accompanied by absent distal pulse, reduction of the fracture/dislocation may return a kinked or stretched artery to its normal position and may relieve the arterial insufficiency. However, reduction should be attempted carefully and the deformity should not be exaggerated in these cases to avoid additional damage to the vessels.
c. A vascular examination must be repeated after any manipulation of the fracture site or whenever the patient develops symptoms that suggest possible ischemia.
d. A distal vascular examination must be done in any proximal open injury which is bleeding profusely.

Management of the vascular injuries involves immediate diagnosis (arteriogram may be performed if indicated) and repair within 6 hours of the injury. When the arterial repair is required, it is best performed by a vascular surgeon. It is

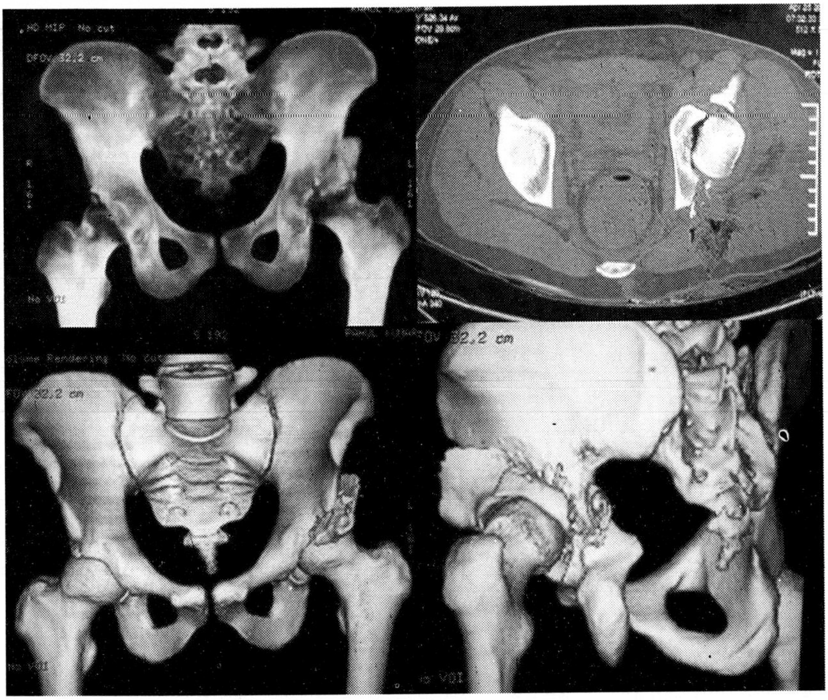

Fig. 5.2: This 20-year-old patient with posterior dislocation of the left hip (Top left: X-rays; Top right: CT scan axial cuts; Bottom: CT scan 3D Reconstruction) presented with sciatic nerve injury. The nerve in these cases can be damaged by stretching, pressure of dislocated femoral head or laceration by sharp fracture fragment. The common peroneal component is most commonly involved in partial injuries

essential to fix the fracture first (usually by plating or the use of an external fixator) to protect the vascular repair. A prophylactic fasciotomy should be done in most cases for possible compartment syndrome resulting from the reperfusion syndrome after the vessels are repaired.

4. **Injury to nerves:** Nerve injuries are relatively uncommon but are commoner than arterial injuries. Nerve injuries may result from traction, impingement or laceration. Nerve injuries associated with closed fractures are usually due to neuropraxia resulting from stretch and resolve spontaneously with time. The treatment is expectant in these cases. However, a cut injury/laceration of the nerve should be suspected if there is a penetrating injury or a compound fracture. These injuries often need exploration and repair. Nerve deficit may sometimes appear after manipulation of a fracture and suggests interposition of the nerve between the fracture fragments and is an indication for urgent exploration.

Common sites of nerve injury are:
- Spinal cord and cauda equina (spinal injuries)
- Axillary nerve, brachial plexus (shoulder dislocation, proximal humerus fractures)
- Radial nerve (in spiral groove—humerus shaft fractures)
- Ulnar nerve (medial epicondyle fracture)
- Posterior interosseous nerve (radial head fractures or dislocation)
- Sciatic nerve injury (hip dislocations) (Fig. 5.2)

- Common peroneal nerve (knee dislocations, fibular neck fractures).

Examination to detect nerve injuries including distal sensations and motor power should be performed in all cases and should be documented in all fracture patients. Progression of the deficit is much more important and is more important indicator of urgency of the treatment than the deficit present when the patient is seen. A careful assessment of the vascular status should be done in all the patients with nerve injuries.

The treatment of the nerve injuries is specific to different regions. The nerve injury may also present late as for example after the open reduction and internal fixation of fracture (e.g. humeral shaft fractures due to stretching of radial nerve while manipulating the fracture fragments to reduce the fracture) or may occur due to engulfment of the nerve by the scarring or the callus around. Only an alert clinician with high index of suspicion will be able to recognize the latter deficits and evaluate and manage appropriately.

5. **Skin loss or damage (Fig. 5.3).**
   Significant soft tissue injuries/skin loss are prone to the development of compartment syndromes, infection and other complications.

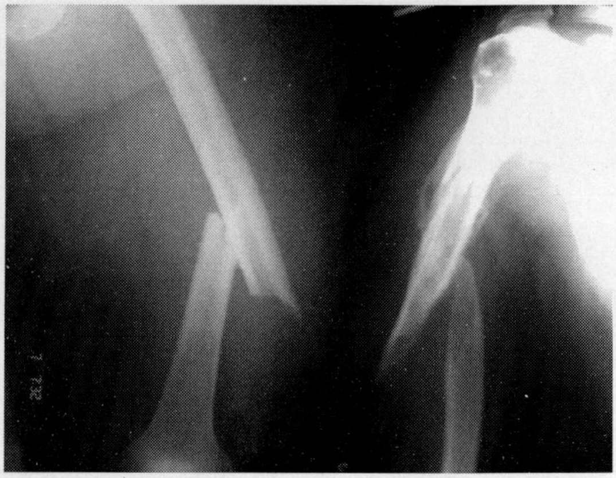

5.3: A sharp spike of fracture fragment (left: femur; right: humerus) can penetrate through muscles or skin and result in compound fracture and/or injury to neurovascular structures

EARLY OR INTERMEDIATE COMPLICATIONS (Table 5.2)

Occur during the period of treatment, within days of sustaining the injury. These complications can be local or general.

Local Complications

1. **Skin or soft tissue necrosis** due to pressure from the underlying bony fragment/dislocated bone or due to vascular compromise. Before skin necrosis, the skin appears blanched and taut and prompt reduction is necessary. Otherwise the skin breaks down and a closed fracture is converted into an open one.
2. **Gangrene** from the vascular injury or external pressure.
3. **Pressure sores** and **nerve palsies** from splintage or traction.
4. **Compartment Syndrome**

Table 5.2: Early Complications of Fractures

Local Complications	General Complications
Skin or soft tissue breakdown	Adult Respiratory Distress Syndrome
Gangrene	Fat embolism
Complicatons due to traction	Tetanus
Pressure sores	Chest infection
Nerve palsies	Disseminated Intravascular Coagulation
Compartment syndrome	Exacerbation of generalized illness
Infections	Deep vein thrombosis and pulmonary thromboembolism
Wound infection	
Gas gangrene	
Necrotizing fasciitis	
Loss of reduction	

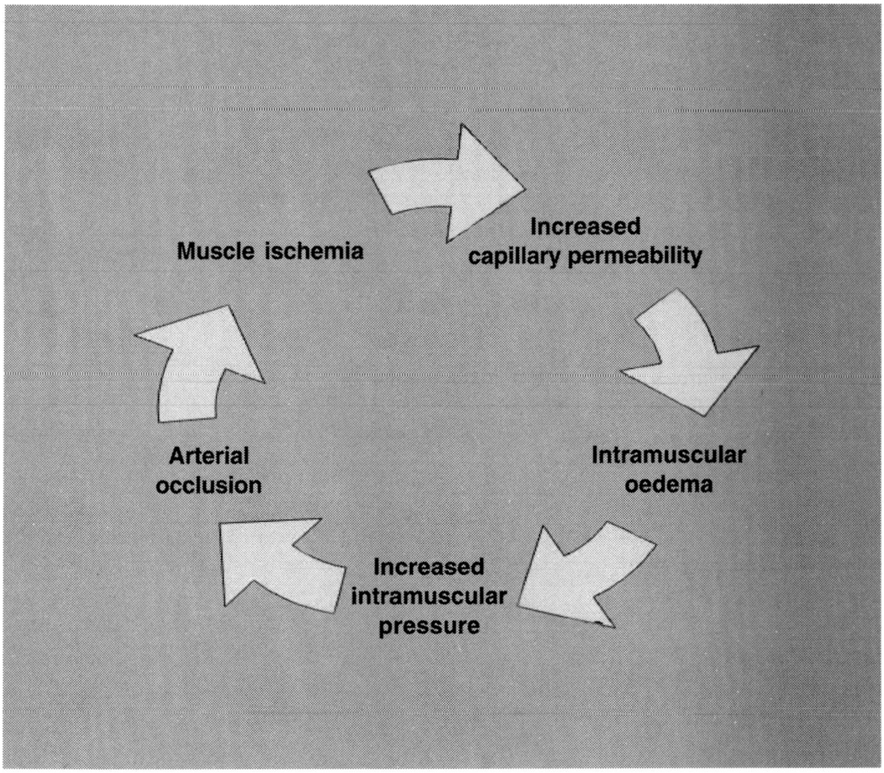

Fig. 5.4A: Pathogenesis of compartment syndrome

Compartment syndrome occurs when the pressure within a rigid fascial compartment prevents adequate muscle perfusion and leads to ischemic tissue necrosis (Fig. 5.4A). It is most common in leg and forearm. Tight bandages are the most common cause of compartment syndrome in our country. Prolonged use of Military Anti Shock Trousers (MAST) also increases the risk.

Clinical features of the compartment syndrome include impairment of two point discrimination (earliest sign). Disproportionate rest pain of injured limb especially with *passive extension of the digits* also occurs early and is one of the most reliable signs. Five "P"s namely Pain, Pallor, Paraesthesia, Paralysis and Pulselessness, when present usually indicate advanced stage and permanent damage and likely loss of the limb.

A high index of suspicion must be maintained to detect this syndrome early. Compartmental pressure measurement must be carried out early in case of suspicion, particularly in patients who are paralysed, unconscious or intoxicated. Whitesides method or electronic indwelling catheter device is used to measure the pressure 5 cm from the fracture site (Fig. 5.4B). Compartmental pressure > 30 mmHg or 30 cm of water or between 10-30 mmHg of the diastolic blood pressure are highly suggestive of the diagnosis.

Treatment consists of removal of all encircling layers on the skin (dressing/casts) and generous skin incision and fasciotomy within 4 hours of onset to prevent muscle necrosis. Necrotic muscle is removed till healthy red, soft, bleeding and contractile muscle is reached.

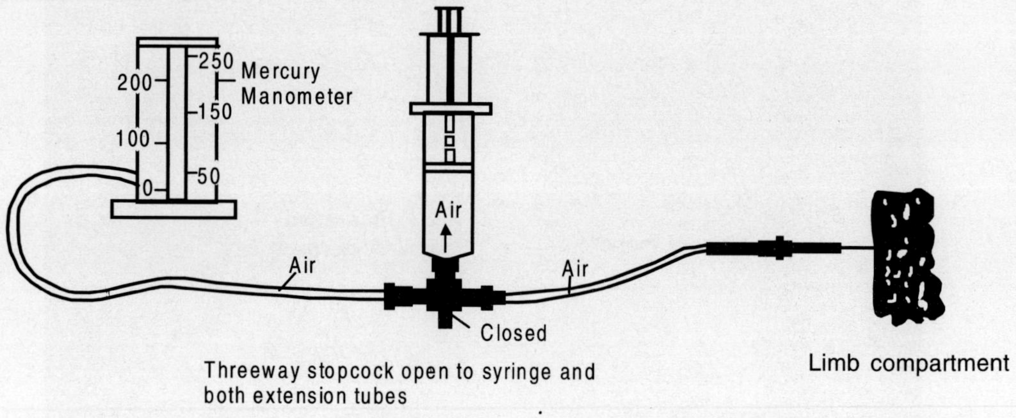

Fig. 5.4B: Whitesides method of compartment pressure measurement. A saline meniscus/air bubble is created in extension tube leading to the affected compartment through a needle. Pressure needed to just move the meniscus equals compartment pressure and is read on mercury manometer connected through the other extension tube

The wound is closed after 4-5 days by secondary closure or skin grafting.

5. **Infection:** Infections occur usually after compound fracture but may also occur after the operative treatment of fractures.
   i. *Osteomyelitis*
   Osteomyelitis can occur following open fractures or internal fixation of the fractures. The important steps in the management of open fractures to prevent infection are:
   - Early surgery
   - Adequate debridement
   - Fracture stabilization
   - Open wound care with early and adequate soft tissue cover
   - Prophylactic antibiotics

   Treatment of chronic osteomyelitis resulting from open fractures depends on the status of the fracture. The aim of treatment in osteomyelitis in the ununited fracture fragments is control of infection (debridement, antibiotics), stabilization of fracture (usually external fixator) and soft tissue flap to obliterate dead space and cover the soft tissue defect. Cancellous bone grafting may be required when there is bone loss and the bed is granulating and healthy. In united fractures with osteomyelitis, the treatment is much like any other chronic osteomyelitis except that the implants should be removed during debridement to expedite control of infection. Careful preoperative assessment, however, must ensure that there is little risk of refracture after implant removal or that the fracture is really united.
   ii. *Gas gangrene:* Gas gangrene is caused by clostridium-a gram positive anaerobe. It occurs following farmyard injury, badly contaminated wound or in the drug addicts. Usually it occurs when the fracture is associated with injuries which penetrate to the muscle. The onset of disease is gradual with little toxemia. Infection presents with pain and wound drainage. The exudate is brown, thin in consistency and foul smelling. The infection typically progresses rapidly to local spread, anaerobic myonecrosis, toxaemia and death. The treatment is prompt surgical decompression and debridement. Large intravenous doses of penicillin (3 million units every 3 hours or 6

million units every 6 hours) should be started. Hyperbaric oxygen is extremely beneficial. Fluid and electrolyte replacement is important. Polyvalcnt tetanus antitoxin administration with 50,000 units every 4 to 6 hours for the next 24 to 48 hours is indicated. The best prevention against gas gangrene includes adequate debridement and prophylactic antibiotics including penicillin and metronidazole.

iii. *Tetanus* is caused by Clostridium tetani. It can occur after open fractures. It may present with local or generalised muscle spasm and muscle hyperirritability and even death. Prevention is by early boosters and toxoid for susceptible injuries. 0.5 ml tetanus toxoid should be given to patients with active immunization. In patients with unknown immunization history or whose immunization has lapsed, 250 units of tetanus immunoglobulins should also be given in the opposite arm.

iv. *Toxic Shock Syndrome:* Occurs due to gram positive bacterial superinfection and can occur sometimes even in benign looking wounds.

v. *Necrotizing fasciitis:* Occurs due to streptococcal infections which can be life threatening, especially in immunocompromized patients. High index of suspicion is crucial and presence of blistering cellulitis and/or crepitus should raise the suspicion. Management consists of early diagnosis, decompression, debridement and treatment with penicillins. Delay in diagnosis is associated with high morbidity and mortality.

6. **Loss of alignment or failure of internal fixation**: The treating physician must decide whether the displacement is acceptable or not.

General Complications

Adult Respiratory Distress Syndrome (ARDS)

ARDS can be caused directly by aspiration or inhalation or indirectly (e.g. due to sepsis, shock) by the severe trauma. The condition is characterized by dyspnea and tachypnea, and reduced oxygenation of arterial blood caused by decreased pulmonary function. Latter is the result of pulmonary edema, increased intrapulmonary shunting and decreased pulmonary compliance and functional capacity. Chest X-ray (Fig. 5.5 Right) and arterial blood gas analysis confirm the diagnosis. The treatment needs admission to intensive care unit and ventilatory support with PEEP.

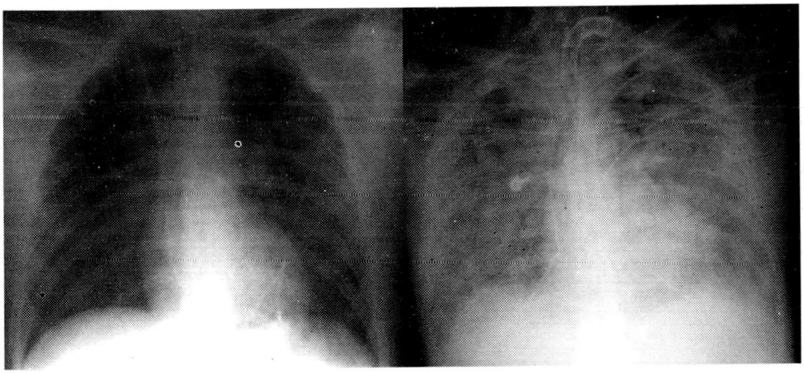

Fig. 5.5: Fat embolism syndrome: X-ray may present as interstitial prominence suggesting interstitial edema (left). In the late stages, the chest X-ray may appear like ARDS (right) with widespread air space consolidation on both sides with confluent soft shadows with fluffy margins; lung bases are involved to greater extent. Air bronchogram is seen. High resolution CT scan shows ground glass appearance

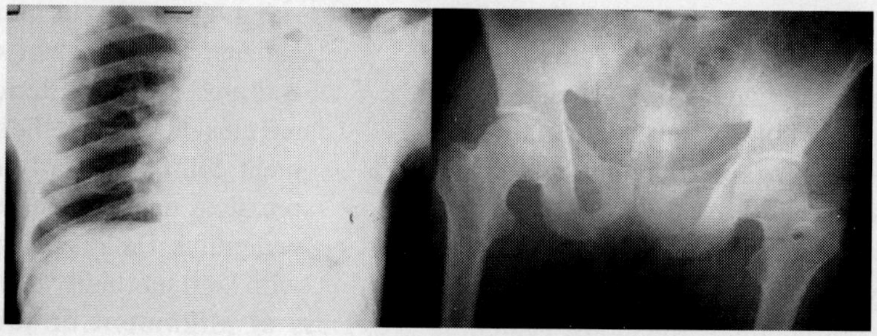

Fig. 5.6: Pneumonitis involving left lung (left). Patient was admitted with pelvis fracture (right)

Fat Embolism Syndrome (FES) leads to hypoxia from pulmonary insufficiency. It results due to systemic release of bone marrow fat and change of chylomicron stability and conversion to free fatty acids in lung parenchyma. It is usually associated with long bone fractures in young adults or hip fractures in the elderly. It may occur in 0.5-2% of patients with multiple fractures. It generally develops more than 12 hours after fracture (Most commonly 24-72 hours after fracture) but may occur even upto 10 days after injury. It usually presents with hypoxia, drowsiness, confusion and restlessness. Other features are tachycardia, fever, tachypnea and oliguria. Changing neurological status is a reliable indicator of the syndrome's onset. Many patients go on to develop petechiae over upper trunk and conjunctivae, go into coma and die. There is no pathognomonic test for FES. Presence of marrow fat in circulation may not lead to FES. Arterial hypoxemia (arterial PO_2 commonly falls to between 60 and 70 mmHg) is the hallmark of FES. Serial X-rays may show evidence of ARDS at a later stage (Fig. 5.5). ECG shows prominent S wave, arrhythmia, inversion of T-wave and right Bundle Branch Block (BBB). The platelet count is low. The serum lipase is raised. Fat globules may be present in the urine. Treatment is supportive. Fractures of long bones should be stabilized early (within 24 hours) to prevent the occurrence of FES. Oxygen therapy is the mainstay of treatment. Ventilatory support may be required. Intensive care monitoring is must. Low molecular weight dextran may improve microcirculation and is recommended by some authors. It is contraindicated in patients with pulmonary edema, renal failure, congestive heart failure, or dehydration. Use of heparin which is recommended by some authors as lipolytic agent is controversial. Systemic (Massive does of methylprednisolone—30 mg/kg intravenously) and intratracheal steroids are claimed to be beneficial but their role is not established.

Chest Infection (Fig. 5.6) Chest infection can occur in elderly patients or in patients with lung injury/ARDS. Antibiotics and supportive oxygen are the mainstay of treatment.

Disseminated Intravascular Coagulation (DIC) is caused by formation of microvascular thrombi that consume platelets and clotting factors, resulting in a vicious cycle of an increased tendency to bleed. DIC can follow any injury and is due to a disturbance of the clotting mechanism. Investigations reveal increased value of PT/PTT (Prothrombin Time/Partial Thromboplastin Time), increased serum levels of fibrin degradation products (FDP) and decreased levels of antithrombin III and fibrinogen. Treatment consists of treatment of underlying cause, judicious use of heparin and Fresh Frozen Plasma and platelet transfusions. Intensive care admission is obligatory.

Exacerbation of generalised illness can occur in unfit patients and common examples are diabetes, chest disease, hypertension, coronary insufficiency etc.

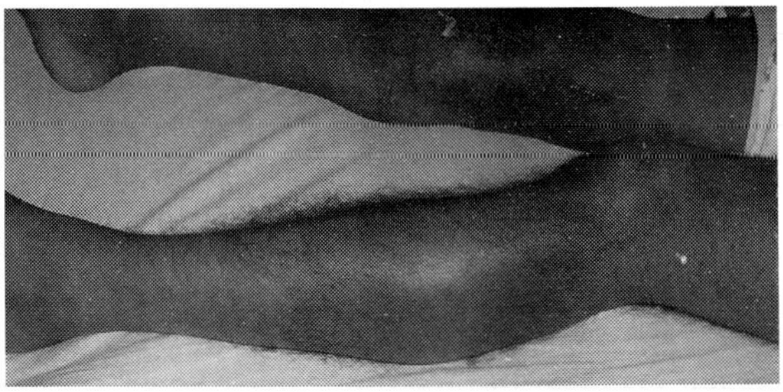

Fig. 5.7: Deep vein thrombosis—Clinical appearance. Remember that the clinical diagnosis of DVT is unreliable

Deep Vein Thrombosis (Fig. 5.7) occurs due to classic VIRCHOW'S TRIAD of injury to endothelium, venous stasis and hypercoagulability. It is especially common after hip fractures, spine fractures with paralysis, pelvis and acetabular fractures and polytrauma. The risk factors include obesity, malignancy, congestive heart failure, varicose veins, contraceptive pills, smoking, immobilization, pregnancy and history of thromboembolism.

Clinical features are unreliable for diagnosis and include calf pain, swelling and fever. Homan's sign may be positive (elicited by passive dorsiflexion of the ankle which causes pain in the calf). Venography is the gold standard for investigations. Other investigations include Duplex ultrasonography (B mode), Radioactive iodine labelled fibrinogen and Impedance Plethysmography. Treatment is by heparin therapy followed by 3 months of warfarin therapy. Oral anticoagulant therapy is monitored by PT testing periodically. Prophylaxis is the most important factor in decreasing morbidity and mortality and includes prevention of immobilization, pressure stockings or pneumatic compression and LOW MOLECULAR WEIGHT HEPARIN.

Pulmonary Thromboembolism (PTE) occurs in 0.2% cases with DVT and can be fatal. It presents with pleuritic pain, tachypnea and tachycardia. Chest X-ray is usually normal. ECG shows right bundle branch block pattern, right axis deviation, ST segment depression and T wave inversion.

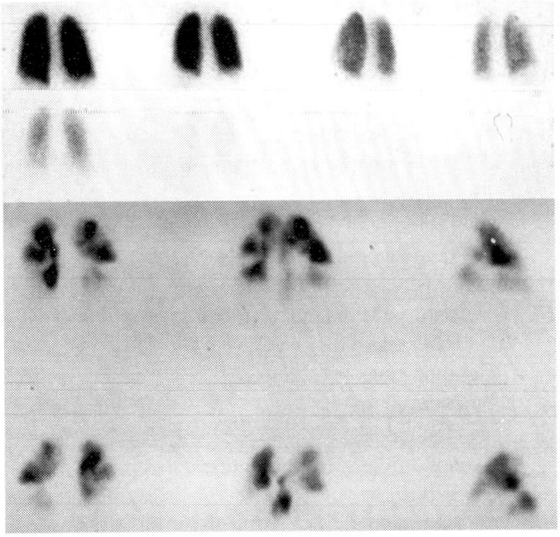

Fig. 5.8: V/Q scan for pulmonary embolism showing ventilation perfusion mismatch. Ventilation scan (Top) shows uniform distribution of xenon gas. Perfusion scan with Tc99 mc (Bottom) shows significant areas without perfusion

Arterial blood gas shows hypoxemia (low blood PaO_2) but normal PaO_2 does not rule out PTE. Ventilation Perfusion Scan (V/Q scan) shows mismatch in PTE (Fig. 5.8). Treatment consists of heparin therapy monitored by partial thromboplastin time (PTT) which is continued for 7-10 days and then switched to 3 months of oral warfarin therapy monitored by PT and INR (International Normalized Ratio).

LATE COMPLICATIONS (Table 5.3)

Occur late in the course of treatment, often several months after injuries. Late complications can affect soft tissues, skeletal tissue or a part of limb.

Myositis ossificans (Fig. 5.9) An extensive calcified mass appears in the soft tissues near a joint and restricts motion. It is seen most commonly around elbow, but may occur at shoulder, hip and knee joints also. It is very common in paraplegics and following head injury. In acute phase, there is increased temperature, swelling, tenderness and

Table 5.3: Late Complications of Fractures

- *Soft tissues*
  - Myositis ossificans
  - Nerves
    - * Late nerve palsies
    - * Entrapment of nerves in the callus
  - Tendons
    - * Tethering of tendons in the callus/at fracture site
    - * Tendon rupture
- *Skeletal*
  - Deformity (Malunion, shortening, cross union)
  - Avascular necrosis
  - Complications of healing
    - * Delayed union
    - * Non union
  - Complications affecting joints
    - * Stiffness
    - * Posttraumatic osteoarthritis
  - Growth disturbances
- *Involving the whole/part of limb*
  - Reflex Sympathetic Dystrophy

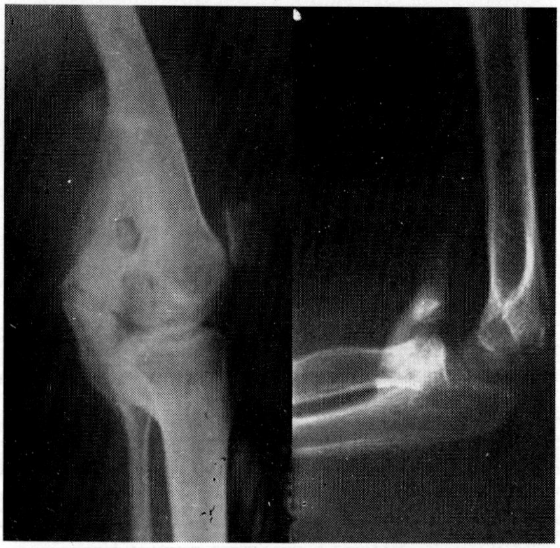

Fig. 5.9: Myositis ossificans following injury to knee (Left) and elbow (Right)

erythema around the joint. Serum alkaline phosphatase (SAP) is raised. X-rays show soft tissue swelling followed by fluffy calcification. Later on (6-12 months later) the local signs suggesting inflammation subside, SAP becomes normal and X-rays show mature bone. Surgical treatment should be undertaken only if the bony mass is interfering with function and should be done only in late stage (after 6-12 months of onset). Recurrences are common and NSAIDs and local radiotherapy can reduce the incidence of recurrence.

Late nerve palsies may appear due to entrapment of the nerve in the fracture callus. Sometimes a nerve palsy may appear several years after injury (**Tardy nerve palsy**) as happens in case of ulnar nerve, when, in the case of cubitus valgus deformity following epiphyseal injury/malunion, the slow stretching of the nerve as it winds around the medial epicondyle leads to tardy ulnar nerve palsy.

Entrapment of tendons may occur due to adherence to the local callus or fibrous tissue at the fracture site or due to malunion (e.g. peroneal tendon entrapment/compression between the lateral malleolus and malunited calcaneal fracture). Tendons may rupture after fractures (as in case of Extensor pollicis longus-EPL-which may rupture after Colles' fracture).

Deformity

Malunion is said to be present when a fracture has united in a clinically significant deformed position. This deformity may be of no consequence as for example fractures of the clavicle almost always unite with a little shortening and overlap but are of no functional or cosmetic importance. However, sometimes malunion interferes with function or is responsible for a poor cosmesis e.g. Dinner fork deformity following Colles' fracture or Gunstock deformity following the supracondylar fracture of the humerus (Fig. 5.10). Malunion may be due to angulation, overriding, malalignment of joint surface or rotation. Malunion with shortening and/or angulation is particularly functionally disabling in the lower extremity fractures. Most cases of malunion are preventable and the initial fracture management is crucial to avoid this complication. Once united, only treatment is an osteotomy to restore anatomical position or

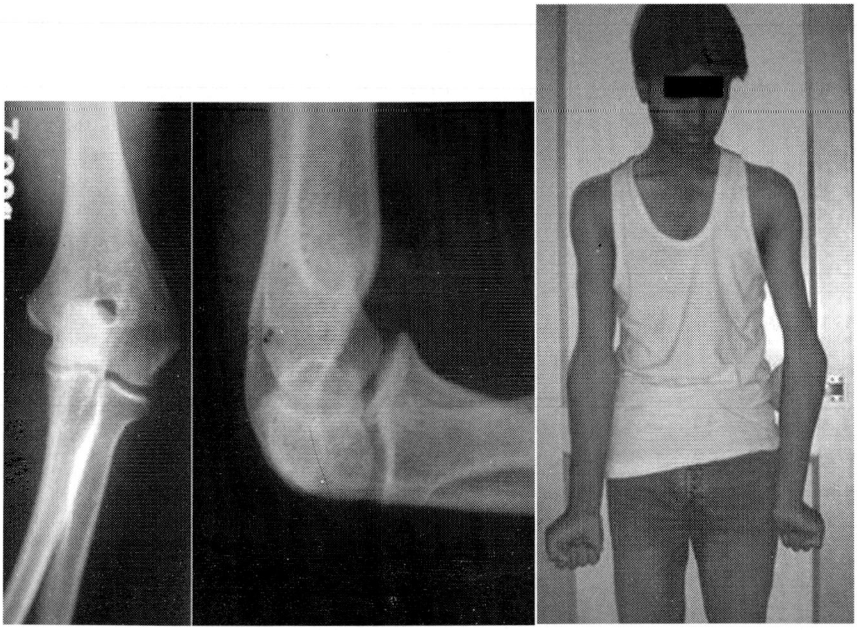

Fig. 5.10: Malunion of supracondylar fracture of humerus resulting in loss of carrying angle (cubitus varus) on left side

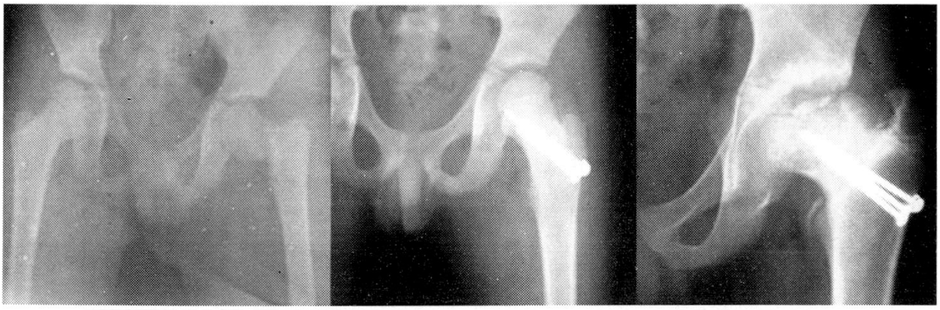

Fig. 5.11: Avascular necrosis of femoral head. Fracture neck femur in a child (left) treated with Moore's pins (middle) with late avascular necrosis (right). Note the loss of contour of femoral head with collapse and sclerosis of femoral head

optimum function and the risks of this procedure must be carefully weighed against possible benefits.

Shortening is functionally important only in the lower extremities. Shortening up to 1 inch (2.5 cm) is compensated well while walking and needs no shoe raise. Shortening more than 4 cm needs limb lengthening.

Cross union occurs when two adjacent bones are united by bridging new bone following fracture. It is particularly disabling in the forearm fractures where it blocks rotations (pronation and supination).

Avascular Necrosis

Avascular Necrosis (AVN) (Fig. 5.11) occurs when disruption in the blood supply due to injury or treatment leads to death of a bone fragment. It leads to non union, collapse and subsequent (secondary) osteoarthritis. The most common site for AVN is femoral head following intra capsular fractures of the neck of femur. Other sites are in the wrist (proximal scaphoid) after scaphoid fracture, in the ankle (Proximal talus) following the talar neck fracture, proximal humerus and femoral condyles. Radiologically the affected bone appears denser than the surrounding bone because the dead bone does not undergo disuse osteoporosis but the surrounding bone does and therefore, gets decalcified. This makes the dead bone appear denser on the X-rays. Also, collapse of the trabeculae and deposition of calcium salts on the dead bone accentuate this dense appearance.

Treatment includes revascularization procedure (local or free vacularized muscle pedicle grafts), excision of avascular fragments, fusion (arthrodesis) or replacement of the joint (e.g. avascular necrosis of femoral head causing pain, stiffness and degenerative secondary osteoarthritis of hip is treated by total hip replacement procedure).

Complications of Healing

Delayed union occurs when the process of union occurs at a rate slower than would normally be expected. Practically, delayed union is said to exist in a fracture that still allows free movement at the fracture site until three to four months after injury. Fractures with delayed union often eventually unite and therefore should be distinguished from non union.

Non union occurs when a fracture fails to unite in the maximum permissible time and shows signs of non-union on X-rays such as closing of medullary cavity, rounding off of the fracture ends and the absence of bridging callus. Clinically, the fractures which are still mobile six months after injury are said to have gone into non union. The causes of non union are listed in chapter 1. The non union can be (i) Atrophic: no visible callus, bone ends tapered off, rounded, osteoporotic and avascular—treated by internal fixation and bone grafting. Union is more difficult to achieve and prognosis is guarded. (ii) Hypertrophic: Hypertrophic callus but non bridging, bone ends are sclerotic, expanded and vascular-treated with internal fixation. Bone grafts are needed only sometimes. Prognosis for union is good (Fig. 5.12).

COMPLICATIONS AFFECTING JOINTS

Stiffness of the neighbouring joint may result after any fracture. The causes for stiffness can be:

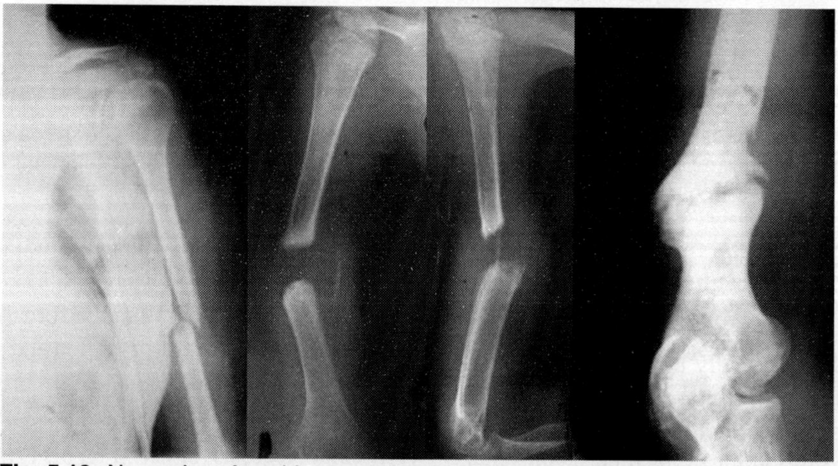

Fig. 5.12: Non union. Atrophic non union humerus (extreme left); Gap non union, a type of atrophic non union, with bony defect in middle; and, hypertrophic non union of humerus (extreme right)

1. Within the joint
   a. Intrarticular fibrous adhesions due to organization of joint hematoma, articular cartilage damage by trauma, or cartilage degeneration due to prolonged immobilization.
   b. Intrarticular fracture leading to irregularity of joint surface, mechanical block or bony loose body.
   c. Secondary osteoarthritis of joint due to malunion, injury to articular cartilage and/or avascular necrosis.
2. Causes close to the joint
   a. Persistent angulation of a fracture leading to altered arc of motion, tethering of muscles/tendons or mechanical block.
   b. Adherence of muscles and tendon to the developing callus e.g. classically seen in adherence of the quadriceps muscles to the site of fracture shaft of the femur.
   c. Contracture of joint capsule
   d. Myositis ossificans
   e. Low grade infections, and
   f. Reflex sympathetic dystrophy.
3. Remote factors
   Such as post traumatic fibrosis of muscles due to vascular injury or compartment syndrome. For example, Volkmann's ischemic contracture of the forearm muscles following supracondylar fracture with vascular injury restricts the wrist and finger joint movements of the ipsilateral hand.

Treatment options for stiffness are limited. Physiotherapy may work early in the course but joint stiffness not responding to physiotherapy is difficult to treat. Manipulation under anaesthesia, excision of myositic mass, release of tethered muscle (e.g. quadricepsplasty for knee stiffness) and lengthening of the contracted muscle can be tried. Stiffness due to intra articular cause can be adressed with arthrolysis or arthroplasty (including joint replacement).

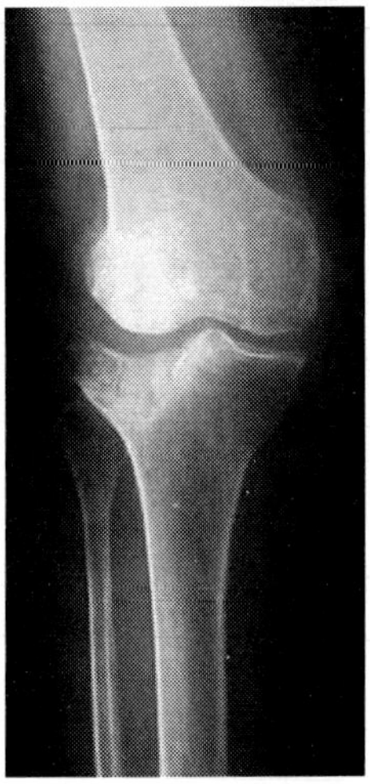

Fig. 5.13: Post traumatic osteoarthritis in the lateral compartment of the right knee due to intra-articular malunited fracture

Post Traumatic Osteoarthritis (Fig. 5.13)

Occurs following intra articular fractures especially with malunion, loose bodies in joint, avascular necrosis and articular cartilage injury. Patient presents several years (or even decades) after injury with pain and restriction of movements with or without deformity. Treatment consists of arthrodesis (fusion of the joint) in young patients or arthroplasty in older patients whenever possible.

Growth Disturbances (Fig. 5.14A, B)

Occur following the growth plate injuries in children. Salter Harris classification (Chapter 1) provides prognostic implications. The children can have limb length discrepancy, angular deformity, joint instability and secondary osteoarthritis. Treatment options include limb lengthening procedures, corrective osteotomy, arthrodesis (in young patients) and arthroplasty respectively.

Reflex Sympathetic Dystrophy (RSD) (Fig. 5.15)

Can occur following trauma or surgery. It results from vasomotor dysfunction of the sympathetic nervous system (sympathetic over activity) in response to pain in a patient who is predisposed

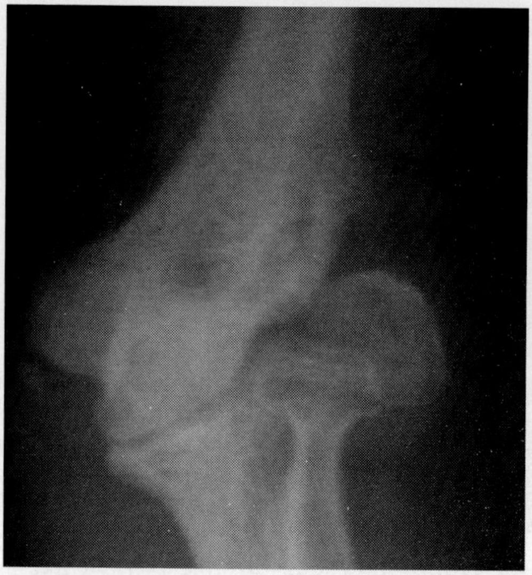

Fig. 5.14A: Growth disturbance of distal humerus due to lateral condylar epiphyseal injury in childhood. Note that the fracture is still ununited

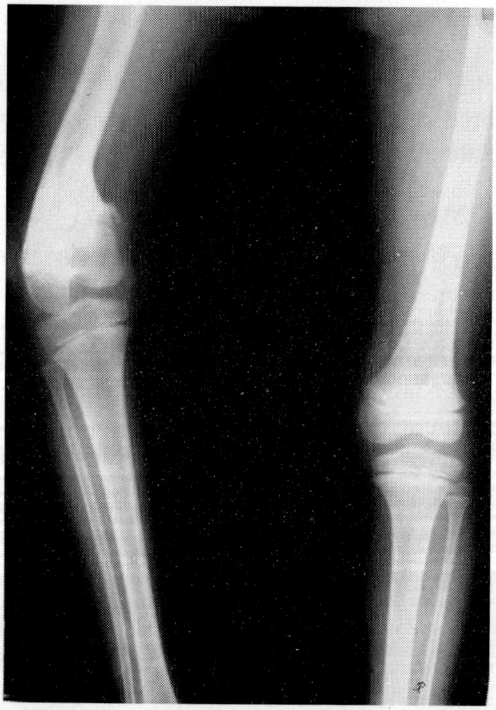

Fig. 5.14B: Growth disturbance of distal femur due to epiphyseal injury. Note that there is angular deformity (genu varum) as well as shortening

because of his personality. Disease presents with pain, swelling, discoloration and stiffness. Disease has three stages:

i. Acute—Characterized by pain, mottled or dusky smooth skin.
ii. Dystrophic—This stage has maximal pain, stiffness and brawny edema
iii. Atrophic—Characterized by skin atrophy, contractures, severe joint stiffness and demineralization. Investigations include triple phase bone scan which shows increased uptake in all the three phases and the diagnostic feature of pain relief by sympathetic block. Treatment consists of adequate pain relief, mobilization of joints by physiotherapy and sympathetic blockade by long acting anaesthetic injection of the stellate ganglion for the upper limbs, or epidural injection for the lower limbs to interrupt the vicious cycle. Prognosis depends on the stage of the disease and gets worse with advance of disease. In mild cases the recovery may be spontaneous while incomplete recovery is the rule in atrophic stage.

FRACTURE EMERGENCIES

Normally fracture emergencies take priority after the ABC's of trauma care. Usually the treatment of a closed or open fracture can be delayed. However the following situations require rapid, decisive action.

1. *Unreduced dislocation of a major joint:* Should be reduced early. Delay in treatment may cause avascular necrosis, nerve palsy, vascular compromise or compartment syndrome. An unreduced dislocation of hip may be the cause of shock, may lead to avascular necrosis and its management takes precedence over Head Injury.
2. *Progressive loss of neurological function following:*
   i. Spinal injury
   ii. Vascular injury with expanding hematoma causing neural deficit by compression. Intervention has to be emergent to prevent

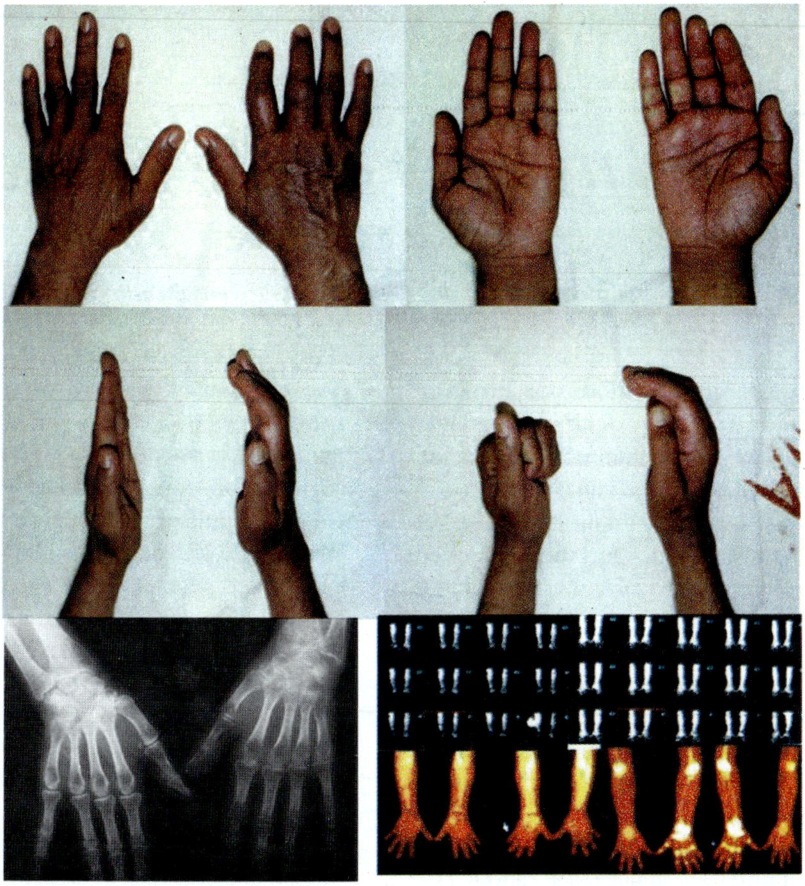

Fig. 5.15: Reflex sympathetic dystrophy (Top and Middle) Clinical pictures showing swelling, discoloration and stiffness of joints. (Bottom) X-ray (left) showing patchy osteoporosis and 3 phase bone scan (right) showing increased uptake in all phases

permanent damage. Progressive loss of neurological function after spinal injury is treated by operative exploration followed by decompression and spinal stabilization. Expanding vascular hematoma is managed by operative exploration with evacuation of hematoma, hemostasis with or without vascular repair.

3. *Compartment Syndrome:* Intervention is urgent to prevent death of muscles and loss of limb function. Immediate operative release of fascial compartments should be undertaken.
4. *Lack of circulation:* Due to injury to vessels by fracture fragments or penetrating injuries. Immediate angiography, exploration and revascularization has to be done to prevent permanent loss of limb function or amputation. Normal function can be restored by prompt action.
5. *Tenting of skin by displaced fragments compromising the vascularity of skin:* As for example, a complete dislocation of talus which can stretch the overlying skin and cause sloughing. Immediate reduction of the dislocation should be performed.

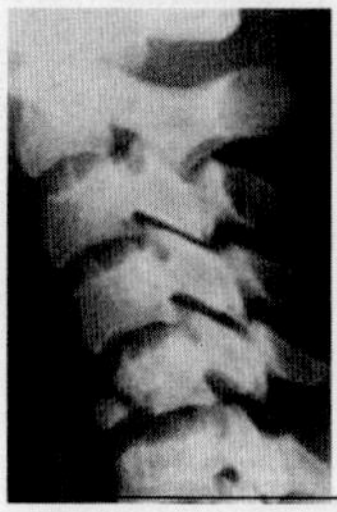

6 Injuries of the Spine

Anatomy, Mechanisms, Clinical evaluation, Classification, Complications, Specific fractures

Injuries of the spine include injuries occurring in the axial skeleton from the occipital–cervical junction to the coccyx. The anatomic classification of the spine injuries is organized into upper cervical, sub axial cervical, thoracic and lumbar, and sacral injuries. Dorsolumbar injuries are more common than the fractures of the cervical spine but the latter are often more serious and may be associated with head injuries. Younger patients fracture their dorsolumbar spine after a high energy force but the fractures in the elderly patients may occur secondary to minimal trauma due to underlying osteoporosis. In fact, in older patients (> 75 years of age), 60% of the vertebral fracutes are caused by falls. About 80% of the patients who suffer from spinal column injuries are males (M:F ratio 4:1).

ANATOMY

- In frontal plane, all segments of spine (cervical, thoracic, lumbar and sacrococcygeal) align in a linear fashion. However, in the sagittal plane, there is approximately 25° of cervical lordosis, 35° of thoracic kyphosis and approximately 50° of lumbar lordosis, thereby allowing the skull to align directly over the mid portion of the top of sacrum. Careful attention must be paid to alignment in the frontal and sagittal planes to identify potential subluxation or dislocation of the spine.
- The spinal cord occupies approximately 35% of the canal at the level of the atlas (C–1) and 50% of the canal in the lower cervical spine and thoracolumbar segments. The remainder of the canal is filled with epidural fat, cerebrospinal fluid and dura mater.
- The segment of the cord from which a nerve root arises lies one level above the same numbered vertebral body until D_{10}.The lumbar segments are concentrated between D_{11} and L_1.
- Conus medullaris is caudal termination of the spinal cord. It contains the sacral and coccygeal spinal cord segments and lies dorsal to the L_1 body and L_{1-2} intervertebral disc. The sacral nuclei which control bladder and bowel function are located in the conus.
- Cauda equina (meaning *horse's tail*) represents the motor and sensory roots of the lumbosacral segments. These roots are less likely to be injured because they have more room in the canal and are not tethered to the same degree as the spinal cord. Also, injuries to the cauda equina are peripheral nerve root injuries and they have a better prognosis for the return of function than do the spinal cord or conus injuries.
- The cross sectional anatomy of the spine is organized into three columns. The anterior column consists of anterior longitudinal ligament, and the anterior half of the vertebral body, annulus fibrosus and disc. The middle column consists of the posterior half of the vertebral body, annulus, and disc, and, the posterior longitudinal ligament. The posterior column includes the facet joints, ligamentum flavum, posterior elements and interconnecting ligaments (Fig. 6.1).

Spinal Injuries: General Considerations

When presented with a spinal injury, the key questions are:

1. Are there other injuries, including life threatening injuries?

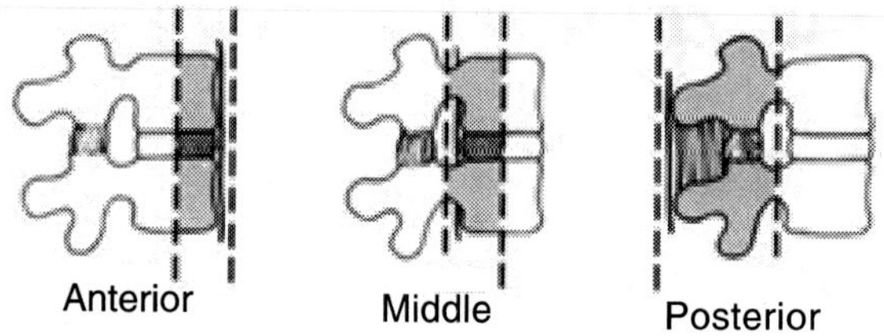

Fig. 6.1: Schematic diagram showing the three columns of spine

2. What is the mechanism of injury?
3. What are the injured anatomic structures in the spine?
4. Is there actual or impending neurologic damage? If the neurologic deficit is present, is it complete or partial cord injury? Is the neurologically injured patient in spinal shock or is the spinal shock over?
5. Can the spine function as a weight bearing column?
6. What is the best treatment method for the particular fracture?

The concept of stability of the spine clarifies the issues of the structural integrity of spine and susceptibility to the neurologic injury.

A **stable spinal injury** is the one which is not associated with the present and future problems of pain, deformity and/or neurological deficit. The spine in these cases can function as weight bearing column.

An **unstable spinal injury** is the one which is associated with actual or potential risk of progressive pain, deformity and/or neurological deficit. An unstable spine is unable to function adequately as a support column and to protect neural elements (acutely and/or chronically). When only one column is injured, the spine is usually stable. When two or three columns are injured, it is usually unstable. An unstable spine is dangerous for it may damage the spinal cord at the time of injury or even subsequently.

Mechanisms and Types of Spine Injuries

Compression fractures are caused by flexion injuries and are characterized by the failure of only anterior column in compression. The vertebral body becomes wedge shaped (Fig. 6.2). These fractures are usually stable. However, when the loss of anterior height is more than 50% of the posterior height, these injuries are unstable.

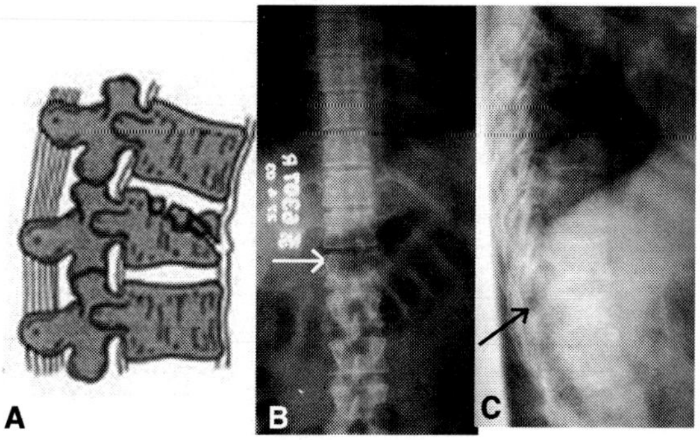

Fig. 6.2: Compression fracture (A) Schematic diagram (B) X-rays AP view of compression fracture of D_{12} (C) Lateral view

Burst fractures are caused by axial loading and are characterized by failure of the anterior and middle columns (Fig. 6.3A-C). They are usually unstable as a result of retropulsion of bony fragments into the spinal canal (Fig. 6.3D).

Seat belt type of injuries are caused by flexion–distraction injuries and are characterised by failure of the middle and posterior columns (Fig. 6.4A, B).

Whiplash or extension distraction injuries are caused by hyperextension and are characterised by the failure of the anterior and middle columns in distraction. It occurs in the rear car collisions (especially if the occupants do not have head restraints) and involves the cervical spine. These injuries are common in patients with cervical spondylosis (Fig. 6.5).

Fracture–Dislocations are characterised by involvement of all three columns in compression, distraction, rotation, and/or shear. These are highly unstable injuries (Fig. 6.6A-E).

CLINICAL EVALUTION OF SPINAL INJURIES

The evalution of spinal injuries must always follow the protocol given below:

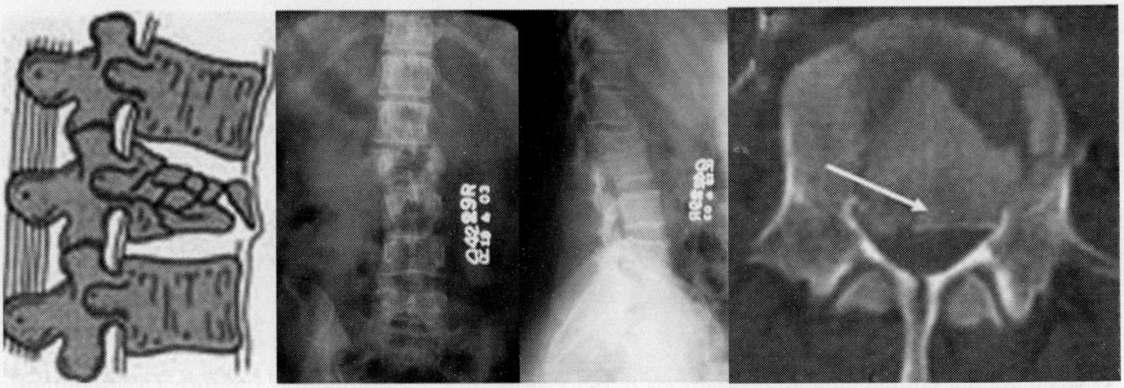

A B C D

Fig. 6.3: Burst fracture (A) Schematic diagram (B) X-rays AP view of burst fracture of L2 (C) Lateral view (D) CT scan axial cut: Note the retropulsed bony fragments in the canal (arrow)

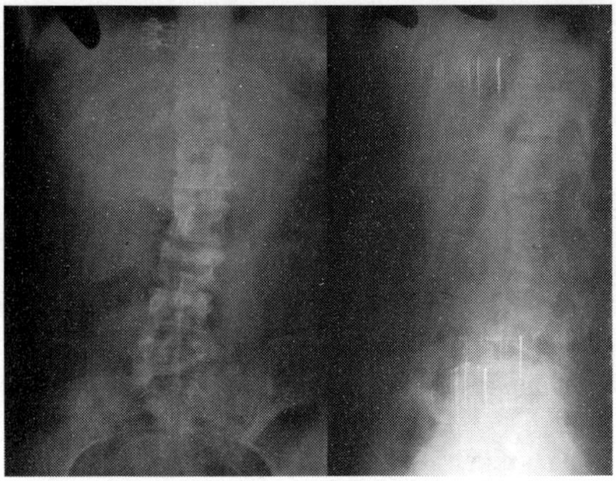

Fig. 6.4A: Chance (seat belt) fracture L2-L3 X-rays—AP and Lateral views

1. Assess the patient: Airway, Breathing, Circulation, Disability.
2. Initiate resuscitation: Address life threatening injuries.
3. Evaluate level of consciousness (Glasgow Coma Scale)
4. Evaluate injuries to head, chest, abdomen, pelvis and spine. Log roll the patient to assess spinal column. Examine skin for bruising and abrasions; palpate spinous processes for tenderness, alignment and diastasis. Look for injuries at more than one (non contiguous) levels.

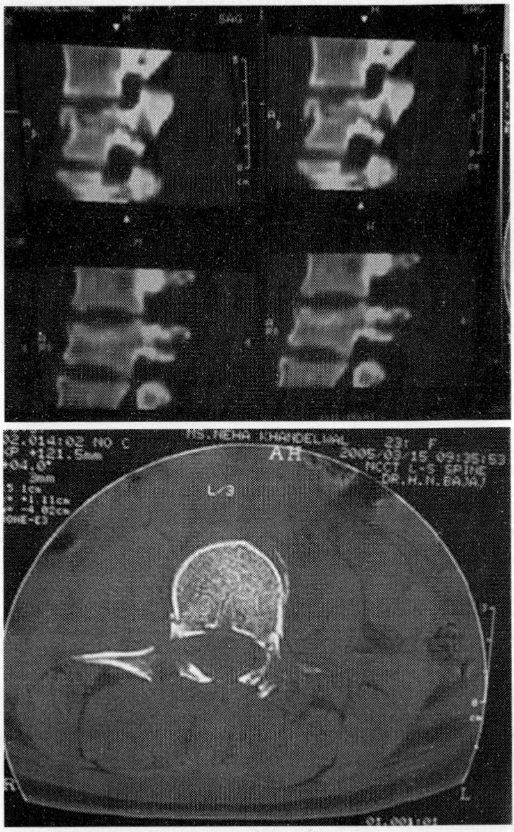

Fig. 6.4B: Chance fracture L2-L3 (Top) CT—Sagittal cut. (Bottom) CT—axial cut. Note the outline of adjacent vertebra on axial cut

5. Assess injuries to extremities.
6. Complete neurologic examination– Motor, sensory (touch, pain, temperature) and reflexes.
7. Perform a rectal examination–perianal sensation, resting tone and bulbocavernosus reflex (S2–3, contraction of anal sphincter in response to the stimulation of the trigone of the bladder with either a squeeze on the glans penis, a tap on the mons pubis, or a pull on the urethral catheter).

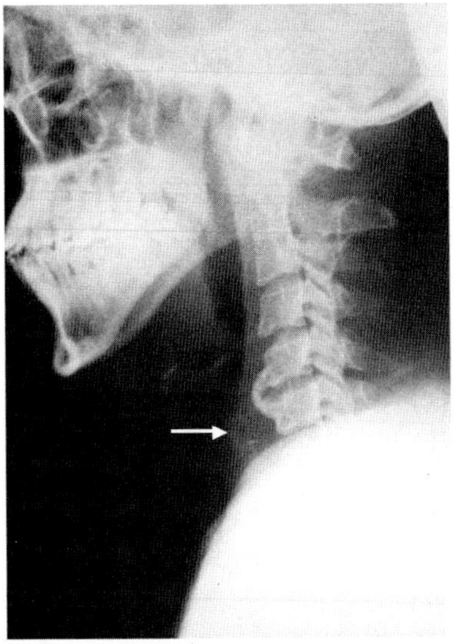

Fig. 6.5: Whiplash injury: Note: Osteoarthritic changes (osteophytes) at C5-C6 in spine and increased prevertebral shadow (arrow). There may be minimal bony changes in these injuries in the form of avulsion fractures from anterior vertebral body or fractures in the lamina

Spinal Shock

Spinal shock is defined as physiological (rather than structural) disruption of the spinal cord function. This phase is classically characterized by the absence of the bulbo cavernosus reflex. Resolution of the spinal shock is recognized when the reflex arcs (e.g. bulbocavernosus reflex) caudal to the level of injury begin to function again, generally within 24 hours of the initial injury. Presence of a complete neurological lesion after the spinal shock has resolved implies a virtually non existent chance of neurological recovery.

CLASSIFICATION OF NEUROLOGIC INJURY

Complete Spinal Cord Injury: is said to be present when there is no sensation or voluntary motor function caudal to the level of the injury in the presence of an intact bulbo cavernosus reflex (indicating resolution of the spinal shock). Reflex activity below the level of cord injury returns. The level of injury is named by the last spinal level

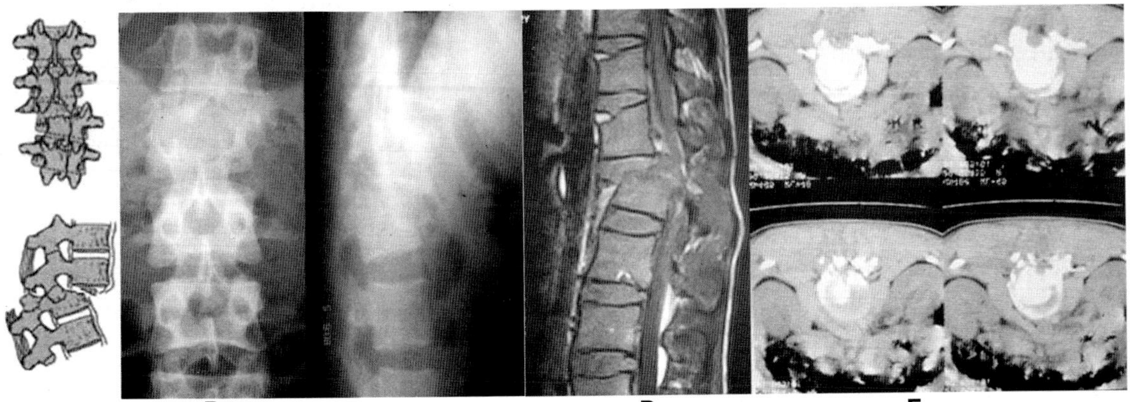

A B C D E

Fig. 6.6: Fracture—Dislocation at the level of L1-L2 (A) Schematic diagram (B) X-rays—AP view (C) X-ray lateral view (D) MRI-Sagittal cuts (E) MRI-axial cuts: Note the compromise of spinal canal and severe cord compression

of partial neurologic function. The prognosis for recovery in these cases is extremely poor.

Incomplete Spinal Cord Injury: is said to be present when some neurologic function persists caudal to the level of injury after return of the bulbocavernosus reflex. *Sacral sparing* is represented by perianal sensation, voluntary rectal motor function and great toe flexor activity and indicates at least partial continuity of the white matter long tracts (Corticospinal and spinothalamic). Sacral sparing indicates incomplete cord injury, with potential for a greater return of cord function after resolution of the spinal shock.

Patterns of the spinal cord injury are shown in Figure 6.7.

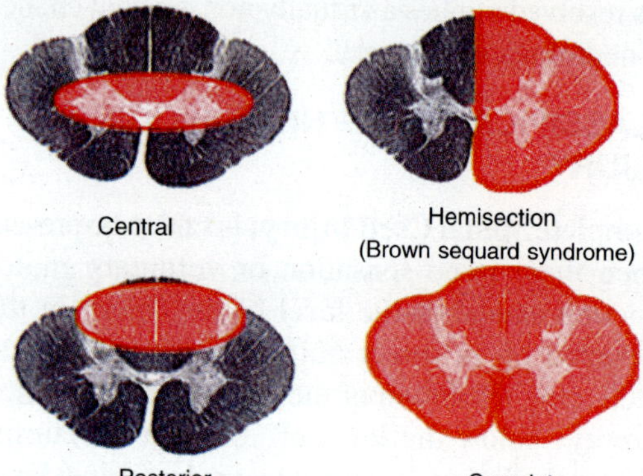

Fig. 6.7: Schematic diagram showing patterns of spinal cord injury

Treatment of Neurologic Injury

1. Immobilization
   - A rigid cervical collar and a backboard in all cases especially with head injury or intoxication. Patient should be moved from the back board only by log rolling maneuver.
2. Radiographic and clinical assessments.
3. Medical Management
   - Methylprednisolone should be given intravenously within the first 4 hours of injury. It may improve the chances of neurologic recovery. It is given in loading dose of 30 mg/kg over one hour and 5.4 mg/kg/hr over the next 23 hours. If the patient presents after 4 hours but before 8 hours after injury, methylprednisoline should be given for 48 hours though the results are inferior. Methylprednisolne should not be given if patient presents more than 8 hours after injury.

COMPLICATIONS OF NEUROLOGICAL INJURY

1. Gastro intestinal
   Ileus, regurgitation, aspiration, hemorrhagic gastritis.
2. Urologic
   Urinary tract infections.
   A paralysed bladder can be automatic or upper motor neuron type (UMN–Injury above S_2, automatic involuntary emptying, no residual urine) or autonomous (lower motor neuron type–injury below S_2, emptying voluntary by manual pressure, large residual urine).
3. Pulmonary
   Pooled secretions, atelectasis, pneumonia.
4. Skin pressure sores (Fig. 6.8).
5. Reflex dysautonomia.

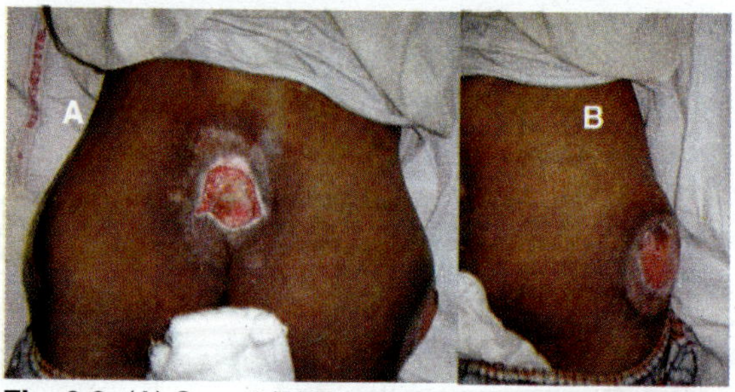

Fig. 6.8: (A) Sacral (B) Trochanteric decubitus sore in a patient with paraplegia

Injuries of the Cervical Spine

Injuries of the cervical spine may occur due to fall from height, diving, road traffic accident (RTA) or gunshot injuries. Cervical spine injuries are commonly associated with head injuries and the neurological damage may be seen in 40% patients with cervical spine injuries. Therefore, *all patients with head injury and all unconscious patients following RTA must have X–rays of the cervical spine.*

Conscious patients usually give the history of trauma following which there is pain, swelling and inability to move the neck with or without weakness of the limbs. Examination reveals tenderness over the involved spinous processes and sometimes, a palpable gap. The neurological examination must document a functional level and the presence or absence of the perianal sensations in addition to the sensory, motor and reflex examination of the extremities.

In suspected cervical spine injuries, the neck must be immobilised with cervical collor or pillows/ sandbags on both sides of the neck.

Radiography of cervical spine injury includes the anteroposterior and lateral X-rays. Latter is more important to diagnose fractures as well as dislocations. Special views may sometimes be required if the routine x–rays are normal.

- Open Mouth View (Fig. 6.9) for injuries of craniovertebral junction, Odontoid fractures, and rotatory subluxation of C_1–C_2
- Oblique projection.
- Swimmer's view (Fig. 6.10) to evaluate C_7/D_1 junction.

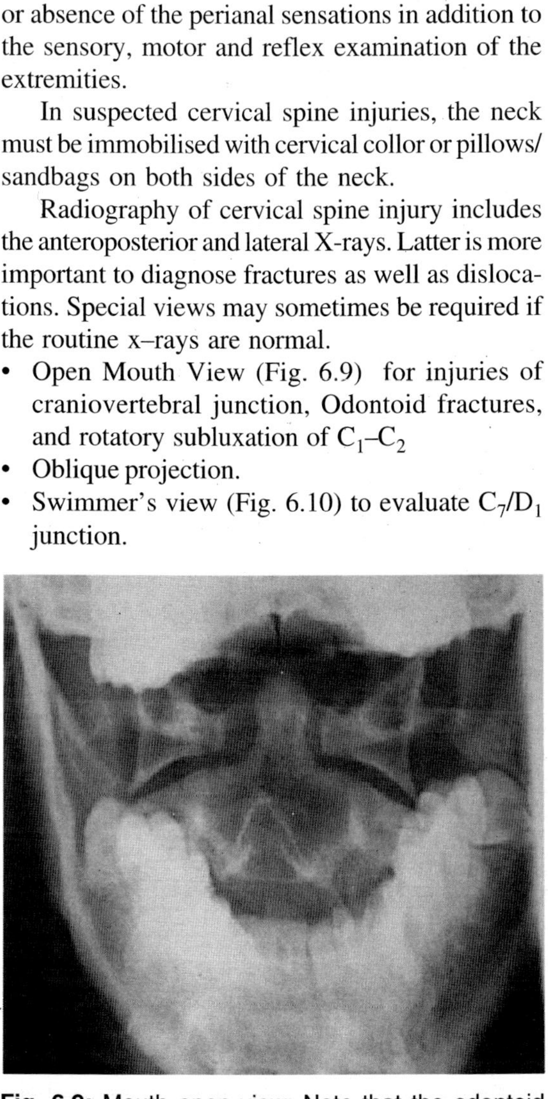

Fig. 6.9: Mouth open view: Note that the odontoid process of C_2 and lateral masses of C_1 are well delineated

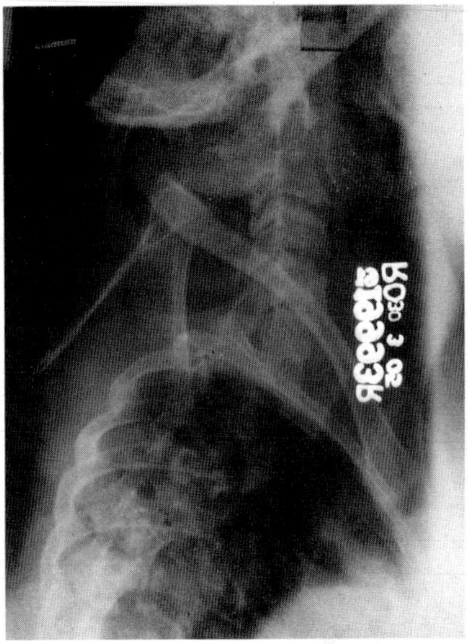

Fig. 6.10: Swimmer's view taken with overhead abduction of one shoulder with other shoulder pulled down to visualize cervico-dorsal junction of spine

Special radiological investigations are sometimes indicated. CT scan makes accurate diagnosis of bony injury including occult fractures and the compromise of the neural canal. MRI evaluates the spinal cord and soft tissue injuries better.

Goals of treatment of cervical spine injuries include resuscitation, safe transport of the patient to hospital (avoiding the so called "Second–accident") preventing further neurological damage, realignment of the spine and aid neurological recovery, achievement and maintenance of spinal stability, early functional recovery and rehabilitation for the residual neurological deficit.

Treatment in cases of cervical spine injury without neurological deficit is non operative. Stable cervical spine injuries are treated in a rigid cervical brace (Fig. 6.11) or Minerva jacket for 8–12 weeks. Unstable cervical spine injury without neurological deficit is treated with skull (skeletal) traction using Crutchfield tongs or Gardner–Wells tongs for 8–12 weeks (Fig. 6.12). Skeletal traction in these cases realigns the spine and maintains the reduction till healing.

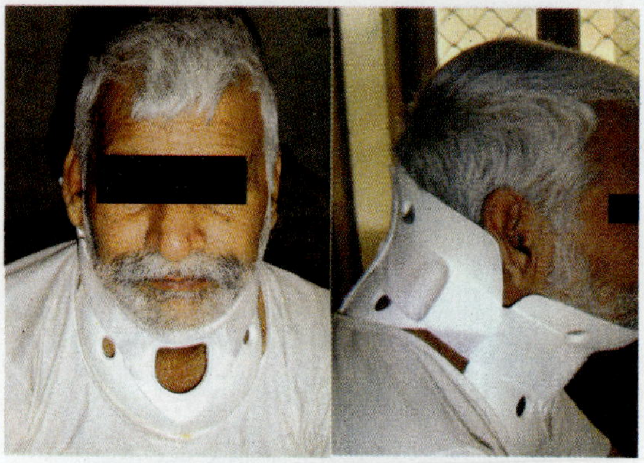

Fig. 6.11: Philadelphia collar

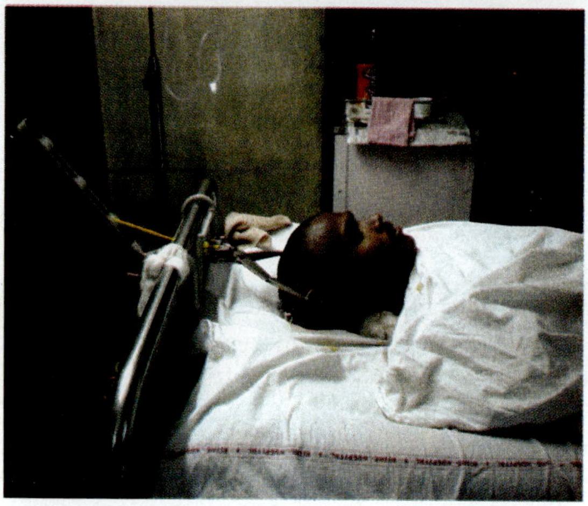

Fig. 6.12: Skull traction using Crutchfield tongs

Treatment of cervical spine injuries with neurological deficit aims to establish the cause and level of the neurological injury (by radiologic assessment) and *urgent* reduction of the unstable bony injury. The skull traction is applied with 10 lb weight for head and 5 lb weight for each subsequent vertebral level till the level of injury with a maximum of 40 lb. Once the reduction is achieved, the weights are reduced by 50 percent and traction maintained for 12 weeks with weekly check X-rays in traction to confirm the maintenance of reduction and regular assessment of the neurological deficit for any improvement/ deterioration.

Surgical treatment is indicated in cases of cervical spine injury when there is inability to achieve reduction (e.g. facet dislocations), in cases with burst fractures with cord compression (for removal of crushed vertebral body) and in cases with late instability to achieve stability.

Special Cervical Spine Injuries

Jefferson's Fracture is the fracture of atlas (C_1) caused by axial loading (fall of heavy object on the head). The arches of atlas are fractured and the distance between the lateral masses increases due to displacement. Usually there is no neurological deficit.

Mouth open odontoid view confirms the diagnosis. Treatment is by rigid cervico thoracic brace for three months.

Odontoid Process Fracture

Odontoid fracture can occur through the tip, junction of odontoid process and body of C_2 or through the upper part of vertebral body of C_2 . Fracture of the odontoid at the junction of the odontoid process and the body (Fig. 6.13) may lead to instability at C_1–C_2 and need wiring and fusion of C_1–C_2. Stable fractures are treated in cervico–thoracic brace or Minerva cast.

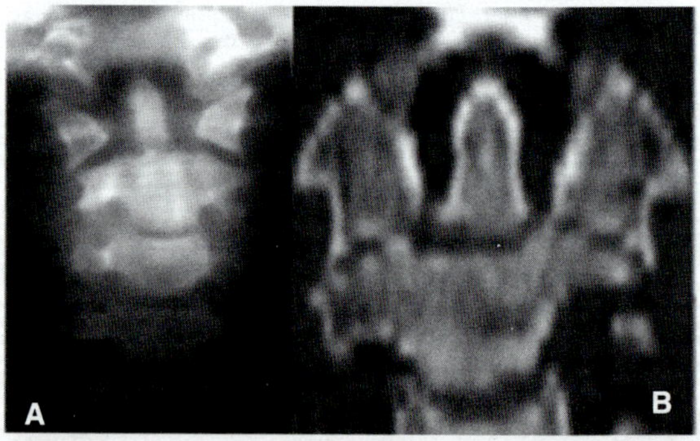

Fig. 6.13: Odontoid process fracture at the base (A) X-ray (B) CT scan

Hangman's Fracture

Hangman's fracture occurs through the pedicle of C_2 with traumatic spondylolisthesis of C_2 over C_3 (slipping forward of C_2 over C_3) due to distraction—extension force as in hanging (Fig. 6.14). Usually there is no neurological deficit and the patient is treated in a rigid Cervico–thoracic brace.

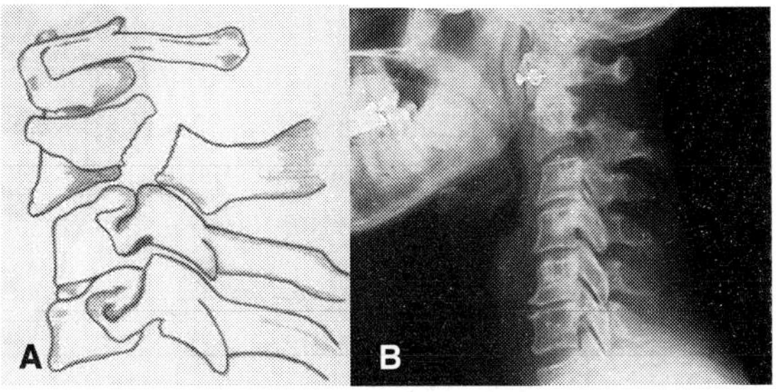

Fig. 6.14: Hangman fracture (A) Schematic diagram (B) Lateral view X-ray

Teardrop fracture is characterised by a triangular tear shaped fracture fragment at the antero–inferior part of the vertebral body (Fig. 6.15).

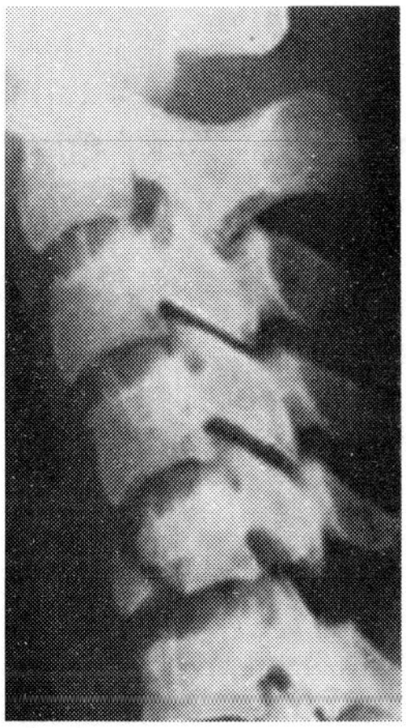

Fig. 6.15: Tear drop fracture C5 vertebra

Subluxation or Dislocation of cervical vertebrae are common in subaxial spine. Pure dislocations are possible only in cervical spine where the horizontal orientation of facets permits dislocation without associated fractures. One (unifacetal) or both (bifacetal) dislocations of the cervical vertebrae can occur (Fig. 6.16). The dislocations compromise the canal dimensions and may lead to neurological deficit. Urgent reduction of the dislocation by skeletal traction is indicated in cases

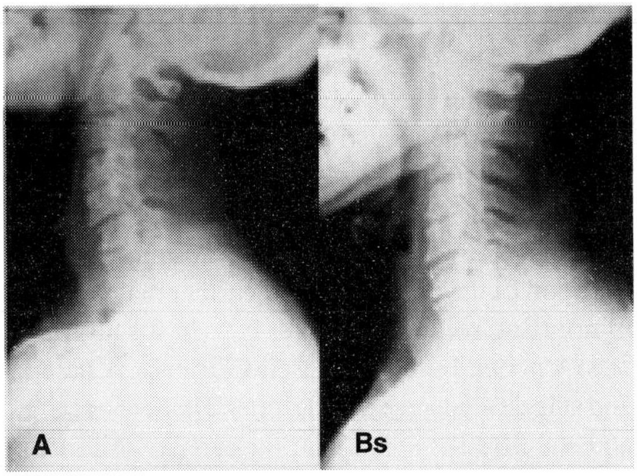

Fig. 6.16: (A) Dislocation of cervical spine at C_5-C_6 level (B) Check X-ray following reduction

associated with neurological deficit. Failure of the dislocation to reduce with skeletal traction is an indication for the open reduction to reduce facetal dislocation.

Injuries of the Thoracolumbar Spine

Thoraco–lumbar area of the spine is the most frequently injured region as it is the transitional area between the kyphotic and immobile dorsal spine and lordotic and mobile lumbar spine. Injuries to this region can occur due to fall from height, road trafic injuries (RTA) and gunshots etc. Fall from height is a common mechanism and may be associated with fracture of the calcaneus bilaterally.

The patient gives history of trauma and complains of pain, tenderness, swelling in the back and/or palpable gap or step between the spinous processes with or without the neurological deficit. Examination is done to document the extent of the neurological damage and the functional level. In all cases of major RTA, spinal injury must be suspected. Conscious patients are asked about the pain in the back and asked to move the limbs voluntarily. Unconscious patients are presumed to have spinal injury till it has been ruled out subsequently. Injury below L_1 presents as cauda equina lesion.

Imaging of the spine begins with the plain radiographs of the spine (AP and lateral) to look for the fracture, disc space and the compromise of the neural canal. CT scan is useful for assessing the bony injury but MRI is the most valuable modality for the investigation of spine injury as it allows accurate visualization of the spinal cord and the soft tissue injury.

Goals of treatment include resuscitation, safe transport of the patient to avoid further neurological injury (Log rolling maneuver is used for all transfers; wooden boards are used to transport patient and at least 4 people should shift the patient), realign and stabilize the spine, aim for early mobilisation of the patient with preventation of the complication of recumbency and the rehabilitation for the residual neurological deficit.

Treatment in cases with stable fracture without neurological deficit includes bed rest for 6–8 weeks, NSAIDs and external support such as corset or plaster jacket.

Unstable fractures without neurological deficit can be treated by internal fixation (usually posterior instrumentation such as, Harrington rods/Hartshill rectangle, Moss-Miami instrumentation) and fusion to allow early mobilisation of the patient, prevent late deformity and/or instability, neurological deficit or pain.

Unstable fractures with neurological deficit are treated with early decompression (anterior, posterior or combined) and spinal fixation (by posterior or combined anterior and posterior instrumentation).

Note: Decompression with or without instrumentation does not improve the neurological recovery. It is recommended primarily to mobilise the patient early to prevent the complications of recumbency. The incomplete and/or neurologically deteriorating cases with compromise of the neural canal and demonstrable compression of cord are the most suitable candidates for spinal decompression.

Common Fracture Patterns

Wedge fracture occurs due to isolated failure of the anterior column due to forwarded flexion. No neurological deficit is seen. Treatment is conservative with rest, NSAIDs and corset/cast.

Burst fracture occurs due to failure of anterior and middle columns. Posterior elements may be intact (stable burst) or injured (unstable burst) with retropulsion of bony fragments in the canal. Neurological deficit and post traumatic kyphosis are common. Decompression and instrumentation to stabilize the spine are recommended for unstable burst fractures.

Chance fracture (Seat belt injuries) occur due to translational injuries sustained by a person wearing seat belt in vehicular accidents. These occur commonly at L_1 level and lead to disruption of all the three columns. Neurological deficit is common. These fractures should be treated by reduction and fixation of the spine by combined anterior and posterior instrumentation.

Fracture dislocations are severe highly unstable injuries with failure of all the three columns and compromise of the neural canal.

Rehabilitation of the Spinal Cord Injured patient

The spinal cord injured patient with significant residual neurologic deficit needs the expertise of orthopedic surgeon, physiotherapist, occupational therapist, rehabilitation experts, psychologist and the social worker.

The treatment aims at minimizing the functional disability by use of orthotics and special appliances. bladder and bowel training with aim to establish reflex emptying of bladder and bowel by techniques such as intermittent catheterization or intermittent clamping of catheter and suppository stimulation of the bowel, bed sore management, physiotherapy and occupational therapy (for modified original or alternative employment). In addition, these patients need sexual rehabilitation, psychotherapy to prevent and treat depression and the social support with encourgement.

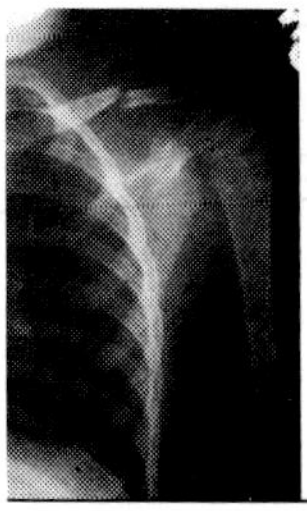

7 Injuries of Shoulder Girdle and Arm

Clavicle, Scapula, Acromioclavicular joints, Shoulder dislocations, Humeral neck, Shaft humerus

The most common injuries in this region are fracture of clavicle, dislocation of shoulder, fracture of the neck of humerus and the fracture of the shaft of humerus. The first step in evaluating these injuries is inspection which often can diagnose these injuries. Brachial plexus injuries may be associated with these injuries and must be looked for. Careful palpation along the clavicle, acromion, coracoid, scapula and humerus to detect tenderness, crepitus or deformity is performed. Painful injuries around the shoulder do not allow the patient to abduct. However, keeping a hand on the deltoid while asking the patient to abduct the shoulder allows the examiner to feel the contraction of deltoid and rule out axillary nerve injuries.

Cardinal features of common injuries around shoulder are summarised in Table 7.1.

Stiffness is commonly associated with these injuries and may involve shoulders but sometimes, hand, wrist and elbow as well. One of the key goals of treating these injuries, especially in the elderly is to preserve movements.

FRACTURE OF THE CLAVICLE

Fracture of the clavicle is one of the most common fractures. More than three-fourth of the fractures involve the middle third which is the weakest area as the cross section of clavicle changes from prismatic in proximal third to the flattened shape of the distal third.

Mechanism of Injury

Fractures of the clavicle occur via direct trauma to the shoulder and occasionally by the fall on the outstretched hand.

Table 7.1: Cardinal Features of Injuries Around Shoulder

Pathology	*Age*	*Trauma*	*Symptoms*
Clavicle fracture	Childhood and early adult life	Fall on outstretched hand or on point of shoulder	Pain, tenderness, swelling, deformity and crepitus at the fracture site
Acromioclavicular dislocation	Young	Fall	Point tenderness at AC joint with or without swelling and deformity
Rotator cuff tear	Middle aged	Fall	Passive movements full: absence or reduced power of active abduction and external rotation
Dislocation of shoulder	Young and middle aged	Abduction and external rotation	Normal fullness gone, pain, increased supero-inferior dimensions of axilla, inability to touch opposite shoulder with hand (anterior dislocation)
Surgical neck of humerus fracture	Old age	Trivial fall	Deformity, pain

Displacement(s)

The outer (distal) fragment is pulled down by the weight of the arm and medially and the inner (medial) fragment is held up by the sternocleido-mastoid muscle.

Clinical Features

A lump is usually obvious. Occasionally a sharp fragment may threaten the skin. Injury to brachial plexus may be present. Injuries to the subclavian artery and vein or internal jugular may occur. Pneumothorax occurs in 3% of cases. Associated injuries to rib cage and rest of the skeleton should be looked for in polytrauma cases.

X-rays: Fracture is usually in the middle third of the bone and the outer fragment lies below the inner (Fig. 7.1). Sterno clavicular or acromio clavicular joint dislocations may be associated.

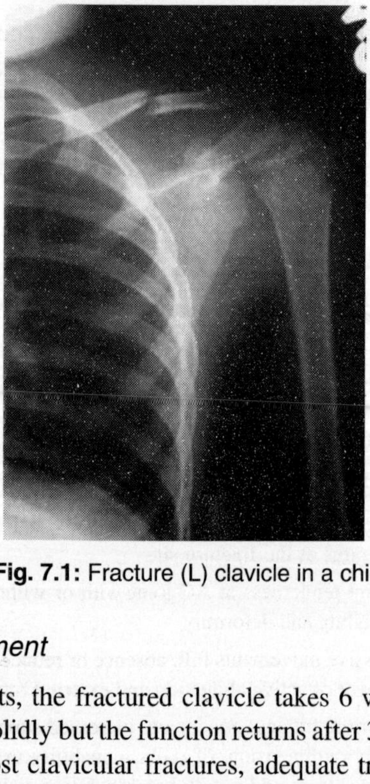

Fig. 7.1: Fracture (L) clavicle in a child

Treatment

In adults, the fractured clavicle takes 6 weeks to unite solidly but the function returns after 3 weeks. For most clavicular fractures, adequate treatment consists of supporting the weight of the arm in a broad sling for the relief of pain. The time honoured method of holding the shoulders braced back by a figure-of-eight bandage has now been discarded as accurate reduction is neither possible nor essential. Tightly applied bandages on the other hand, can constrict and injure the nerve trunks in axilla or obstruct venous return from the upper limbs. Moderate persistent displacement does not hinder union or function and should be accepted.

As soon as the pain begins to subside, active shoulder exercises should be started to restore full mobility. Three weeks of support is normally sufficient.

Surgical treatment by open reduction and internal fixation (most commonly plating) is rarely required and is indicated if there is associated neurovascular compromise, widely displaced fracture fragments with tenting of skin by the fractured ends or open fractures. Symptomatic non unions are treated by ORIF and bone grafting.

Complications

1. Malunion: Most common complication. It is more of cosmetic than functional problem. Deformities soon remodel in children.
2. Neurovascular sequelae: Injury to brachial plexus, subclavian vessels or internal jugular vein.
3. Pneumothorax: Rarely the dome of pleura may be penetrated by a bone fragment leading to pneumothorax.
4. Non union: is rare and seldom causes symptoms. If symptomatic it is treated by internal fixation and bone grafting.
5. Stiffness of the shoulder occurs especially in old persons if the exercises are not started early.

FRACTURE OF THE SCAPULA

Fractures of the scapula are caused by high energy injuries (Fig. 7.2). Fractures of the scapular body are caused by the direct blow or the crushing force while the neck of the scapula is fractured by a blow or a fall on the shoulders (Fig. 7.3).

Fractures of the scapula are rarely displaced and heal rapidly as the scapula is surrounded by

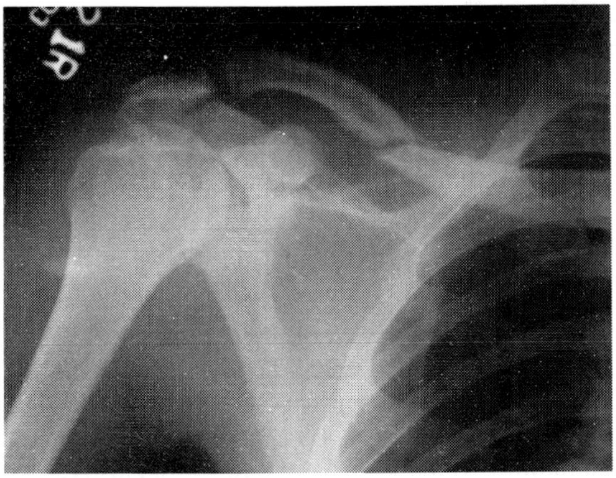

Fig. 7.2: Fracture of the acromion and glenoid of the scapula. Also note the fracture clavicle. This injury typically resulted from high energy trauma

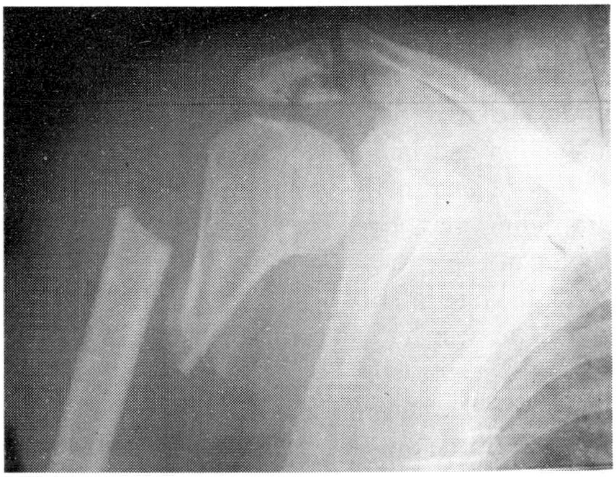

Fig. 7.3: Fracture of the scapular neck, body and acromion. Also note the comminuted fracture of the proximal third of humerus

highly vascular musculature which aids in the rapid healing of the fracture sites.

Fractures of the scapula are of little significance. However, they may be associated with fractures of the ribs.

Treatment consists of simple support in a broad sling with early movements when the pain allows. Surgery is indicated only in fractures through the glenoid which can lead to either instability or osteoarthritis of the shoulder joint. Screw fixation of glenoid fragment usually suffices.

SUBLUXATION AND DISLOCATION OF ACROMIO CLAVICULAR JOINT

Dislocation or subluxation of the acromio-clavicular joint is usually caused by a severe fall on the point of the shoulder and sometimes by a fall on the outstretched hand. The clavicle is normally held in position by two sets of ligaments, the acromio-clavicular ligaments and the coraco-clavicular ligaments. Tearing of acromio clavicular ligaments leads to upward subluxation of the clavicle while more severe injury tears the coraco clavicular ligaments also and leads to dislocation of joint. In both cases, the displacement is difficult to reposition but function is usually good even without reduction of the displacement.

Clinical Features

The patient presents with acute tenderness and swelling over AC joint. The outer end of the clavicle is abnormally prominent and tender. Shoulder movements are restricted. Brachial plexus injury must be looked for and ruled out.

X-ray

Anteroposterior X-rays demonstrate the displacement of the clavicle (Fig. 7.4). If there is doubt, opposite (uninjured) AC joint can be X-rayed for

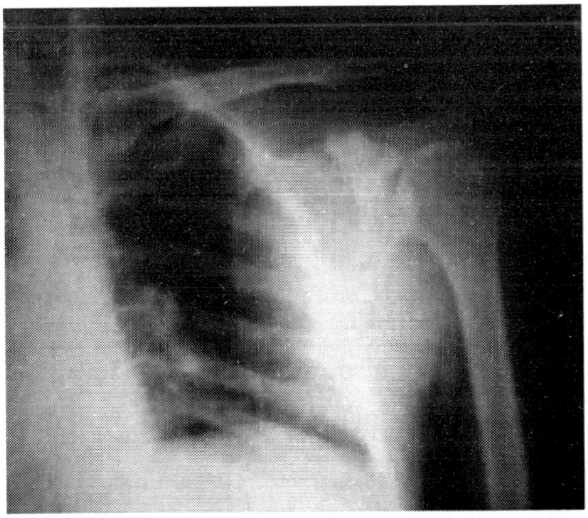

Fig. 7.4: Dislocation of acromio-clavicular joint

comparison. The displacement may be more obvious if the patient holds a weight in hand on the injured side.

Treatment

A broad sling is often sufficient. Shoulder exercises are begun when the pain subsides (usually after 1 week). The subluxation will usually persist but the function is likely to be normal. Rarely, especially in athletes, surgical treatment is undertaken to reduce and hold the clavicle in place. Surgical repair or reconstruction of the coraco-clavicular ligaments is performed and protected by driving a screw from the clavicle into the coracoid process or by passing a mersilene tape around the clavicle and coracoid process. Shoulder is immoblised for three weeks and then exercises are started.

Complications

1. Persistent displacement of clavicle with cosmetic 'bump'.
2. Osteoarthritis of acromioclavicular joint. It occurs late and can be treated conservatively. If marked pain persists, lateral end of the clavicle can be resected.

DISLOCATION OF THE SHOULDER JOINT

Shoulder is the most common site for dislocation as the socket of the shoulder (glenoid) is relatively flat and the stability of the joint is greatly dependent on the surrounding soft tissue structures.

Mechanism of Injury and Types

Anterior dislocation is caused by an external rotation of an abducted arm, as occurs after a fall or motor vehicle accident or during contact sports. Posterior dislocations typically occur following severe trauma and can also occur following falls, car accidents, or epileptic fits.

Most shoulder dislocations are anterior (84%). Posterior dislocations are next commonest. Inferior and superior dislocations are rare.

Clinical Features

Diagnosis is usually easy in anterior dislocations because of the flattening of the deltoid muscle which produces a straight drop in the line of the shoulder from the tip of the acromion (Hamilton Ruler sign). Patient presents with severe pain and supports the arm with the opposite hand. The affected shoulder is typically held in slight abduction and external rotation. The humeral head may be palpable below the coracoid (most common) or in the axilla. A careful neurovascular examination with attention to axillary nerve integrity is performed by feeling for deltoid contraction, while asking the patient to attempt abduction. The musculocutaneous nerve integrity is assessed by the presence of sensations on the anterolateral forearm.

Posterior dislocation is more difficult to diagnose as the abnormality in the contour of the shoulder is less obvious. These dislocations are often missed. The patient presents with arm in adduction and internal rotation with inability to abduct or externally rotate the arm. There is a protruding mass over the posterior aspect of the shoulder.

In the rare inferior dislocations, called Luxatio erecta, the arm lies in a vertical position along side patient's head.

X-ray: The humeral head in anterior dislocation usually lies below and medial to the socket and there are overlapping shadows of the humeral head and glenoid (Fig. 7.5).

Posterior dislocation produces a 'globular' or 'light bulb' appearance of the upper end of the humerus with a clear space between the humeral head and the glenoid. Axillary views can confirm the direction of dislocation.

Treatment: Reduction, preferably under anaesthesia should be carried out as early as possible. Many methods are available.

Hippocratic Technique

Can be performed by a single person. One (stockinged) foot is placed across the axillary folds

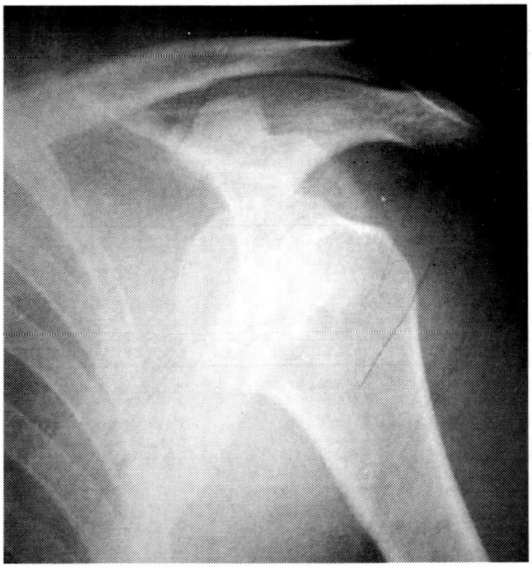

Fig. 7.5: Anterior dislocation of shoulder

and onto the chest wall to provide counter traction. Axial traction is applied on the affected upper extremity with gentle internal and external rotations and the toes slip the head into position to achieve reduction.

Kocher's Method

The humeral head is levered on the anterior glenoid to effect reduction through the sequential maneuvers of (TEA): traction (in abduction), external rotation and adduction. Once the reduction is achieved the arm is internally rotated and immobilised in an arm chest bandage for 3 weeks. This method has high risk of causing fracture of the humerus.

Stimson Technique

After administration of analgesics and/or sedatives, the patient is placed prone on the stretcher with the affected upper extremity hanging free. Gentle manual traction or 5 pounds of weight is applied to the wrist, with the reduction effected over 15 to 20 minutes.

Milch Technique

With the patient supine and the upper extremity abducted and externally rotated, pressure is applied by the thumb of the physician to push the humeral head in place. For posterior dislocations, the axial traction is applied to the arm and the head is pushed forward while the arm is gently rotated externally.

After reduction of either type of dislocation, an X-ray is taken to confirm the position and the arm is immobilised for 3 weeks in a sling, shoulder immobiliser or arm chest bandage. The shoulder exercises are started at the end of this interval.

Complications

1. *Neurovascular injury:* Injury to the axillary nerve and/or artery may occur.
2. *Recurrent anterior dislocation:* This is the most common complication. It is common at younger age, within first two years of the first injury and in males. If the glenoid labrum has been damaged or detached (Bankart lesion), then recurrent dislocation is likely. If the patient is disabled because of recurrent dislocation, surgery is indicated. For recurrent anterior dislocation, Putti Platt (double breasting and shortening of subscapularis) is usually successful. Other commonly performed operations are reattachment of labral detachment (Bankart repair) and transfer of the coracoid process with its muscle attachments to the glenoid rim (Bristow procedure).
3. *Bony lesions*
   a. Hill-Sach's lesion: is a postero lateral humeral head defect caused by an impression fracture on the glenoid rim. It is seen in 27% of acute anterior dislocations and 74% of recurrent anterior dislocations
   b. Glenoid lip fracture: also called "Bony Bankart lesion"
   c. Fracture of Greater tuberosity
   d. Fracture of acromion or coracoid.

4. *Soft tissue injuries*
   a. Rotator cuff tears
   b. Capsule or subscapularis tears.

FRACTURES OF THE HUMERAL NECK

Proximal humeral fractures comprise 4% to 5% of all fractures, and represent the most common humeral fractures (45%). These fractures occur frequently in old patients, more often in females than males due to osteoporosis. A stiff shoulder is a common occurrence.

Mechanism of Injury and Types

These fractures are frequently sustained from low energy trauma as in fall on outstretched hand in elderly and high energy trauma as motor vehicle accidents in younger patients.

Proximal humerus fractures can be undisplaced or displaced, abducted or adducted types, fractures through greater (Fig. 7.6A) or lesser tuberosity, anatomic (Fig. 7.6B) or surgical neck (Fig. 7.6C) or these can be comminuted.

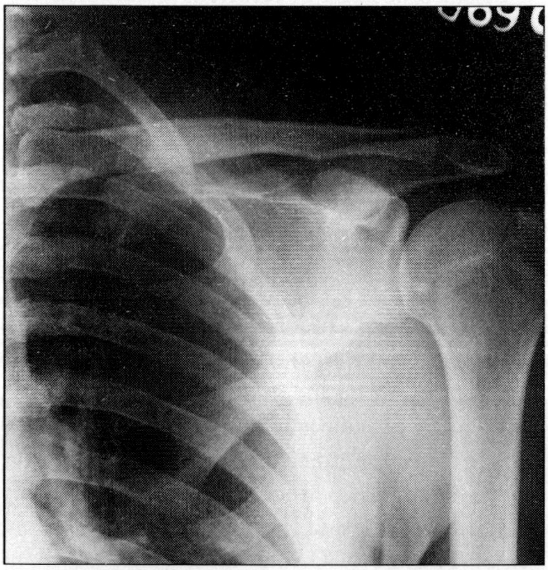

Fig. 7.6A: Fracture of greater tuberosity. This fracture is treated conservatively in a sling with early range of motion exercises

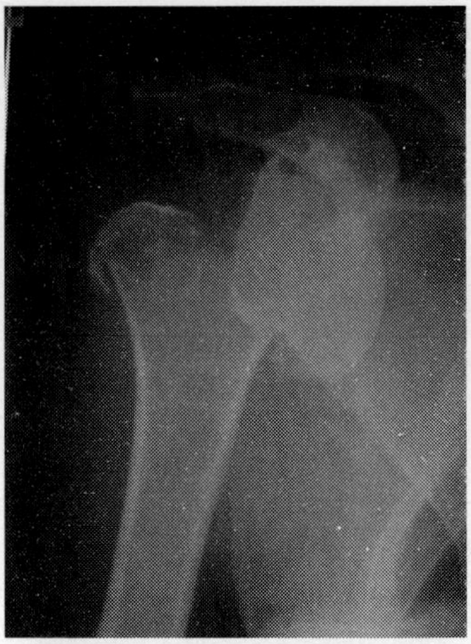

Fig. 7.6B: Fracture of proximal humerus through the anatomic neck. (Also note the minimally displaced fracture of the greater tuberosity

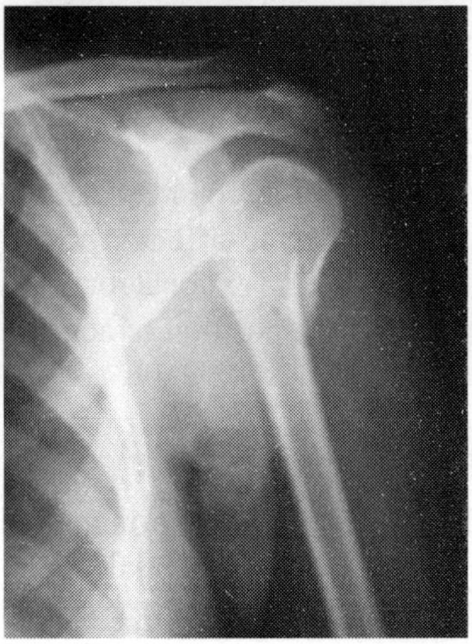

Fig. 7.6C: Fracture of the proximal humerus through the surgical neck

Displacements

The various fragments following the proximal humeral fracture displace according to the muscle attachments:

- The greater tuberosity is displaced superiorly and posteriorly by the supraspinatus and external rotators (muscle attachments on the greater tuberosity can be remembered by SIT—Supraspinatus, Infraspinatus and Teres minor from anterior to posterior).
- The lesser tuberosity is displaced medially by the subscapularis.
- The humeral shaft is displaced medially by the pectoralis major.

- The proximal fragment is abducted by the deltoid insertion.

Clinical Features

Patient typically presents with the upper extremity held close to chest wall, supported by the other hand. There is local pain, swelling, tenderness, painful range of motion and sometimes, crepitus. Ecchymosis may be present on the chest wall and flank and must be differentiated from the thoracic injury. Axillary artery (especially in older patients with calcified vessels) and brachial plexus injuries (especially axillary nerve) may occur and must be looked for.

X-ray

Anteroposterior view demonstrates the fracture and displacements. However, an axillary view is invaluable for associated dislocations and glenoid articular fracture.

Treatment

Most (nearly 85%) of these fractures do not need any operative management. Minimally displaced fractures are treated with sling immobilization (Fig. 7.7). Early shoulder mobilization is started in undisplaced fractures, as early as possible, usually within a few days. Closed reduction and pinning can be done if it is possible to manipulate and reduce the fragments under anaesthesia (Fig. 7.8). Open reduction and internal fixation is indicated for widely displaced tuberosity fractures, severely displaced fractures which are irreducible by closed means and fracture dislocations.

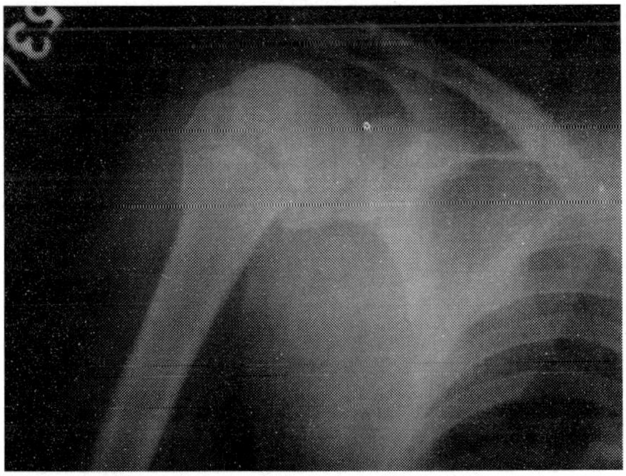

Fig. 7.7: Undisplaced fracture surgical neck of humerus. These fractures are treated non surgically

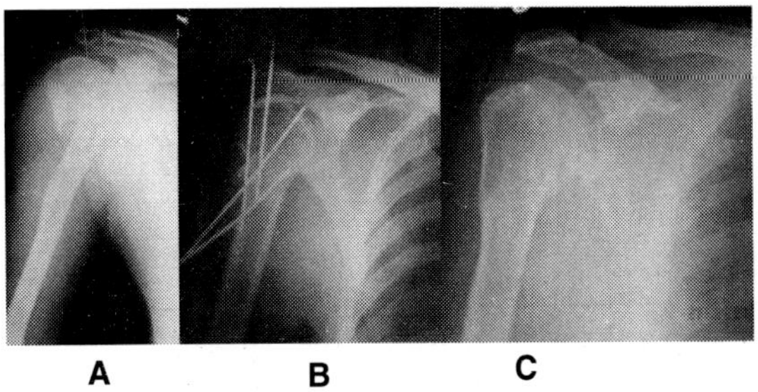

Fig. 7.8: Displaced fracture neck of humerus treated by percutaneous pinning (A) Preoperative; (B) Post operative check film; (C) Final follow up after union

Complications

1. Injury to neurovascular structures. Axillary artery injury may occur in 5% to 6% cases and may occur especially in older patients with atherosclerosis due to loss of vessel wall elasticity.
   Note: Radial pulse may be present even in cases with axillary artery injury due to the collateral circulation.
   Axillary nerve injury and rarely, brachial plexus injury may be associated.
2. Stiffness of the shoulder. Stiffness is treated by aggressive supervised physiotherapy.
3. Avascular necrosis of the humeral head may occur in comminuted fractures/fracture dislocations of the proximal humerus and the anatomic neck fractures. It leads to collapse of head, traumatic arthritis of the shoulder and pain. It is treated by prosthetic replacement.
4. Non union is seen particularly in displaced surgical neck fractures with soft tissue interposition. It is treated by open reduction, internal fixation and bone grafting.

5. Malunion: results in stiffness of the shoulder or blocked range of motion.

FRACTURES OF THE HUMERAL SHAFT

Fractures of the humeral shaft occur among all age groups.

Mechanism of Injury and Types

Humeral shaft fractures can be caused by a direct blow (most common-leads to transverse or comminuted fracture) or indirect (twisting injury or fall on outstretched hand-leads to spiral or oblique fracture). Apart from the configuration of the fracture line, these fractures can be classified according to location (upper, mid or lower third); fractures may be closed or open and simple or comminuted.

Displacements

1. Typical displacements occur due to musculotendinous attachments of the humerus.
   a. Fracture above pectoralis major insertion: Proximal fragment is abducted and externally rotated by the rotator cuff; distal fragment is pulled medially and proximally by pectoralis major and deltoid.
   b. Fracture between pectoralis major insertion and deltoid tuberosity:
   Proximal fragment is pulled medially by pectoralis, teres major and latissimus dorsi; distal fragment is pulled laterally and proximally by deltoid.
   c. Fracture distal to deltoid tuberosity:
   Proximal fragment is abducted by deltoid; distal fragment is pulled medially and proximally by biceps and triceps.

Clinical Features

Patients with humeral shaft fractures typically present with pain, swelling, deformity and shortening of the affected arm. Patient holds the injured extremity apprehensively to avoid sharp pain resulting from the movements of the fracture fragments. Examination reveals gross instability with crepitus on gentle manipulation. Careful neurovascular examination should be done especially to rule out injury to radial nerve.

X-rays

Anteroposterior and lateral views should be taken to assess the configuration of the fracture, location (upper, middle or lower third) and the amount of comminution. X-rays of the shoulder and elbow of the same arm should be taken to find associated fractures. Radial nerve entrapment at the fracture site should be suspected if patient with humerus shaft fracture presents with radial nerve palsy and X-rays suggest soft tissue interposition at the fracture site (Fig. 7.9).

Treatment

The goal is to achieve union in an acceptable alignment and to restore function. Algorithm for management of fracture shaft humerus is shown

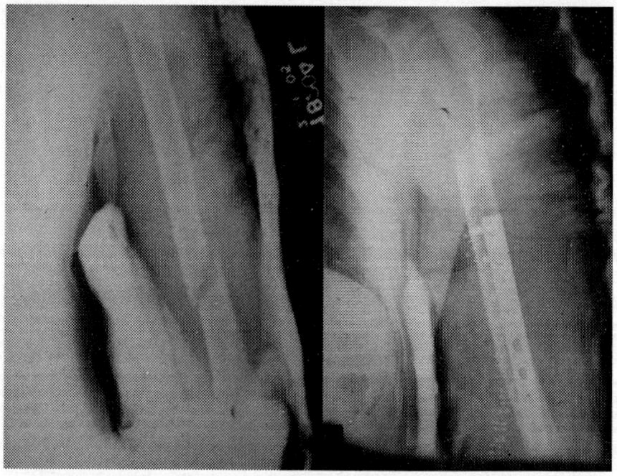

A B

Fig. 7.9: Fracture humerus lower third with radial nerve palsy. Gap at fracture site indicating soft tissue interposition (A) with signs of radial nerve palsy suggests radial nerve entrapment. Treatment consists of exploration of radial nerve—It was found between the fracture fragments in this case—and ORIF with plating for fracture (B)

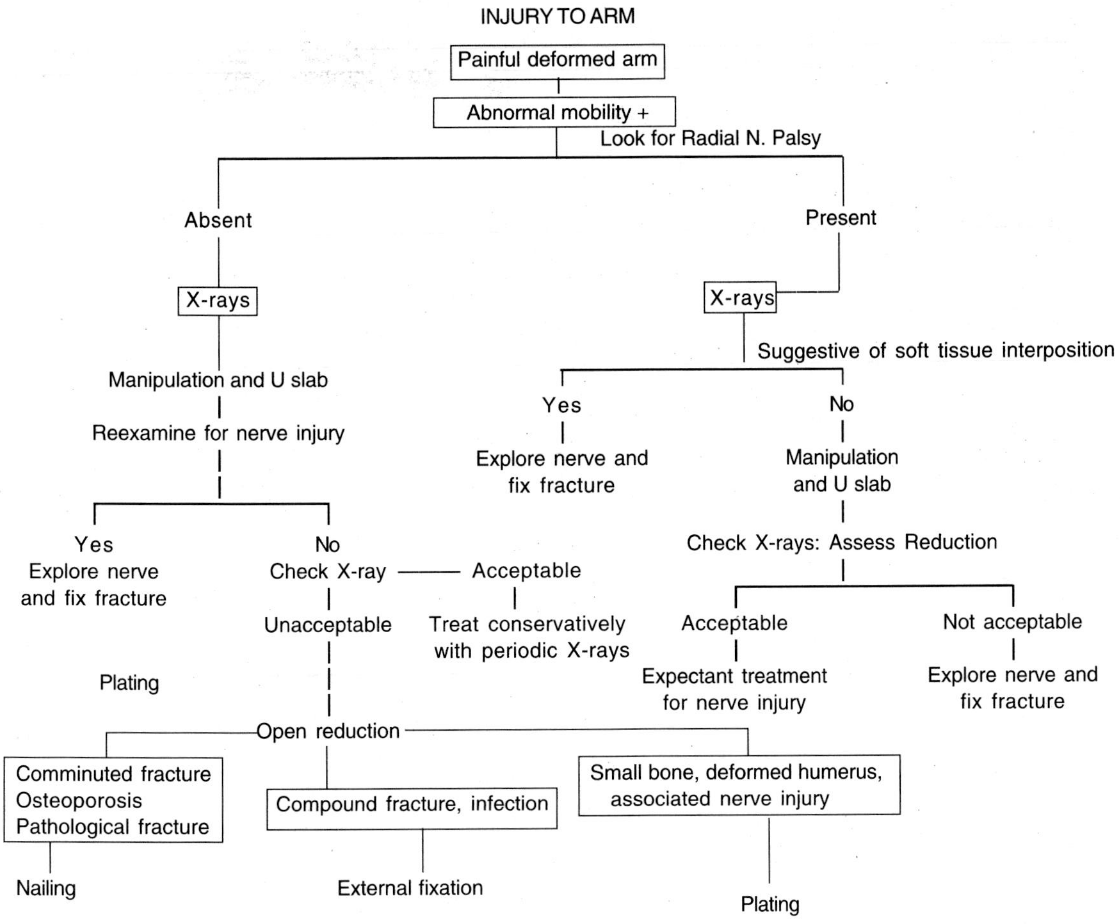

Chart 7.1: Algorithm for management of fracture humeral shaft

in Chart 7.1. Most fractures (>90%) heal with non surgical treatment. Manipulation and U-slab or a coaptation splint application is done and check X-rays taken to assess adequacy of the reduction. Acceptable reduction is upto 20 degrees anterior angulation, 30 degrees of varus and 3 cm of shortening. A hanging cast uses dependent traction from the weight of the cast to effect fracture reduction but may sometimes lead to overdistraction with the risk of non union.

Immobilization may be continued till union (10-12 weeks) or may be exchanged for functional bracing at 1 to 2 weeks. Functional bracing utilizes hydrostatic soft tissue compression to effect and maintain fracture alignment while allowing motion of adjacent joints. It cannot be used in the presence of severe soft tissue injury, for an unreliable patient or when acceptable reduction cannot be achieved or maintained. Functional bracing is continued for 8 weeks after fracture or till the fracture is united radiologically.

Operative treatment of the humeral shaft fracture is to be preferred in patients with multiple trauma, inadequate closed reduction position,

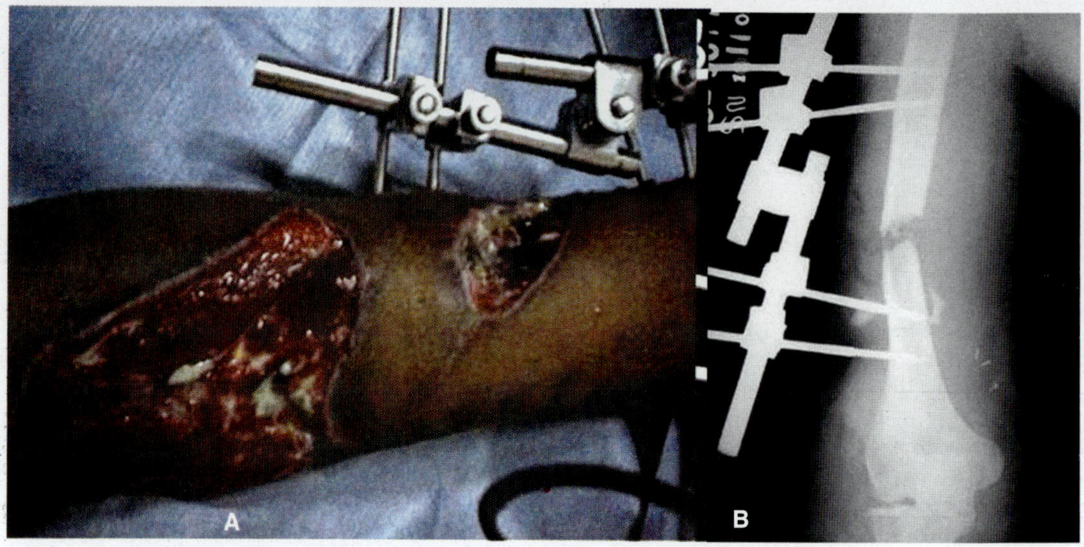

7.10: Compound fracture shaft of humerus with bone loss (A) Immediate treatment consists of debridement and external fixation (B) Bone grafting from the iliac crest has to be done in these cases after 6 weeks to bridge bone gap and enhance union

associated vascular injury, Humeral and both bones forearm fractures in the same limb ("floating elbow"), bilateral humeral fractures, open fractures or neurological (radial nerve) injury following fracture manipulation or penetrating injury. Surgical treatment includes open reduction and plate fixation, closed reduction and locked or flexible intramedullary nailing (especially for comminuted and segemental fractures, osteoporotic bones and pathological fractures) or the external fixation (in the presence of compound fracture with skin or bone loss (Fig. 7.10), burns or infection).

Complications

1. *Neurovascular injuries:* Radial nerve injury may occur in up to 18% cases and is most common after middle third fractures. Most cases (90%) are neuropraxia and function returns within 3 to 4 months. Delayed exploration should be undertaken if no evidence of recovery is seen by electromyography or nerve conduction studies performed at the end of 6 weeks. Laceration is more common in open fractures or gunshot injuries. In these cases, as with palsy

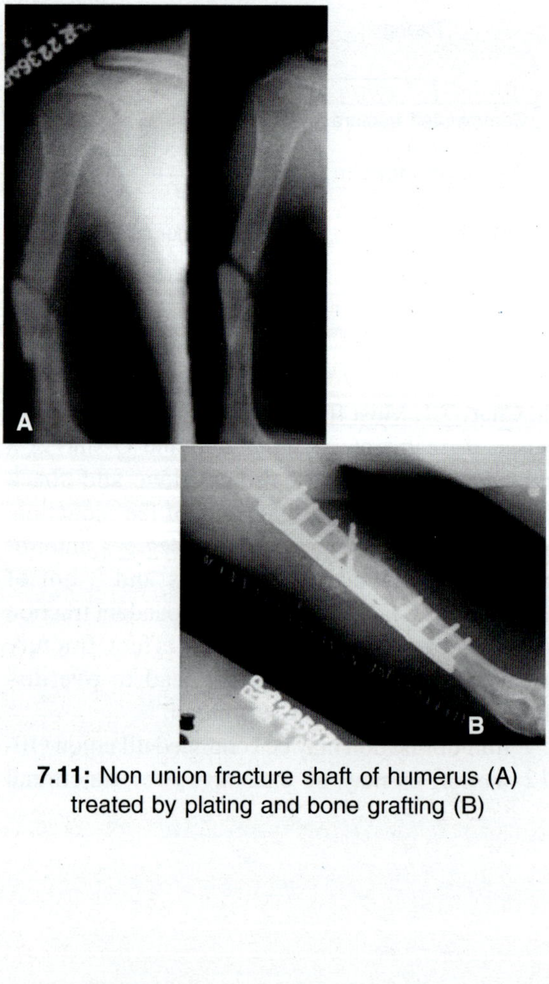

7.11: Non union fracture shaft of humerus (A) treated by plating and bone grafting (B)

appearing after fracture manipulation, early exploration of nerve with fixation of fracture should be undertaken.

2. Non union (Fig. 7.11) may occur in 2-5% patients and is associated with comminuted fractures, soft tissue interposition, inadequate immobilization, high energy trauma with severe bony devascularization and transverse fracture pattern. Treatment is by open reduction and internal fixation with bone grafting.
3. Malunion (Fig. 7.12) may be functionally inconsequential. A large amount of angular and rotational deformity may be tolerated in humerus before it limits the functions as the shoulder is able to compensate for the functional compromise.

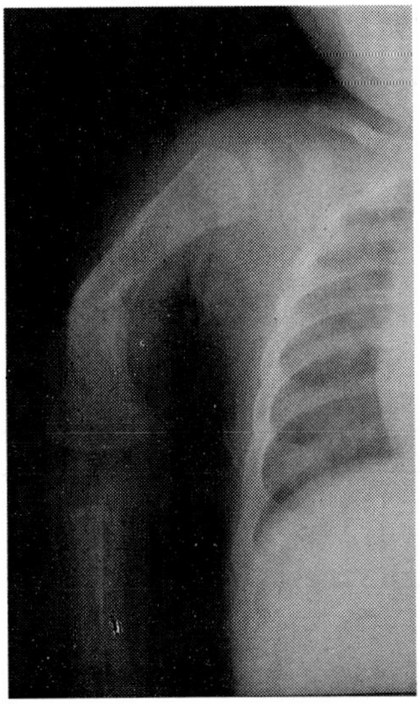

Fig. 7.12: Malunited fracture of humerus in a child. Note the lateral angulation. In children these deformities remodel and treatment consists of observation

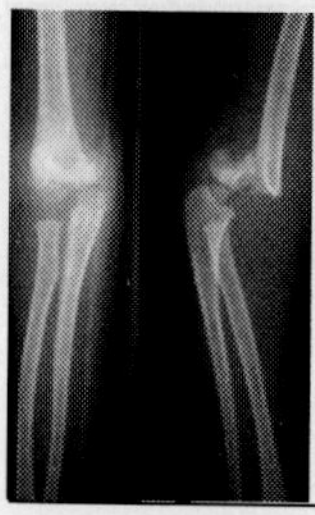

8 Injuries Around Elbow

Supracondylar, Lateral condyle, Medial Epicondyle, Radial head and neck, Intercondylar humerus, Elbow dislocation, Olecranon, Pulled elbow

Elbow fractures in adults and children are among the most complex fractures. Proximity to neurovascular structures leading to high rate of injury and the risk of stiffness lead to poor results. There is a need for near anatomic reduction and early active motion in all intra-articular fractures in this region. Knowledge of normal elbow anatomy and radiographic alignment is essential in diagnosing displacement of fracture fragments.

The injuries around elbow are distinct among the children and adults.The common injury patterns in the two populations are shown in Table 8.1.

The detection of fractures in children is difficult because of the large amount of non ossified cartilage around the elbow. The order of appearance (sequence of the process of ossification) of the various growth centres around elbow can be memorized using the mnemonic CRITOE.

Centre of Ossification	Age at appearance (approximately)
Capitellum	1 year
Radial Head	3 years
Internal (medial) Epicondyle	5 years
Trochlea	7 years
Olecranon	9 years
External epicondyle	11 years

Table 8.1: Common Injury Patterns Around Elbow

Injury	Children	Adults
Supracondylar fracture of Humerus	Common	Rare (occurs only in old osteoporotic patients)
Fracture of the lateral condyle of humerus	Common	Rare
Fracture of the medial epicondyle	Common	Common
Fracture of the radial neck	Common	Uncommon
Intercondylar fractures of humerus	Rare	Common
Fracture of Capitellum	Rare	Common
Dislocation of elbow	Rare	Common
Fracture of the radial head	Rare	Common

Figure 8.1A shows the age of appearance and closure of centres of ossification around elbow. Figure 8.1B shows some of the centres of ossification around elbow in a 6 years old child.

In case of any suspicion the X-rays of the opposite (uninjured) elbow should be taken and compared with the injured elbow. Before obtaining X-rays in children, it is better to splint the elbow in 20 to 30 degrees flexion to relax neurovascular structures and prevent potential injury from sharp fracture fragments. The fractures around elbow may be undisplaced and are often missed on X-rays especially in children. A "Fat pad sign" seen on careful evaluaiton of the lateral film suggests displacement of fat shadow due to bleeding caused by fracture (Fig. 8.2).

Common Fractures of the Distal Humerus in Children

Supracondylar Fracture of the Humerus

More than half of all pediatric elbow fractures are supracondylar. Supracondylar area is the weakest

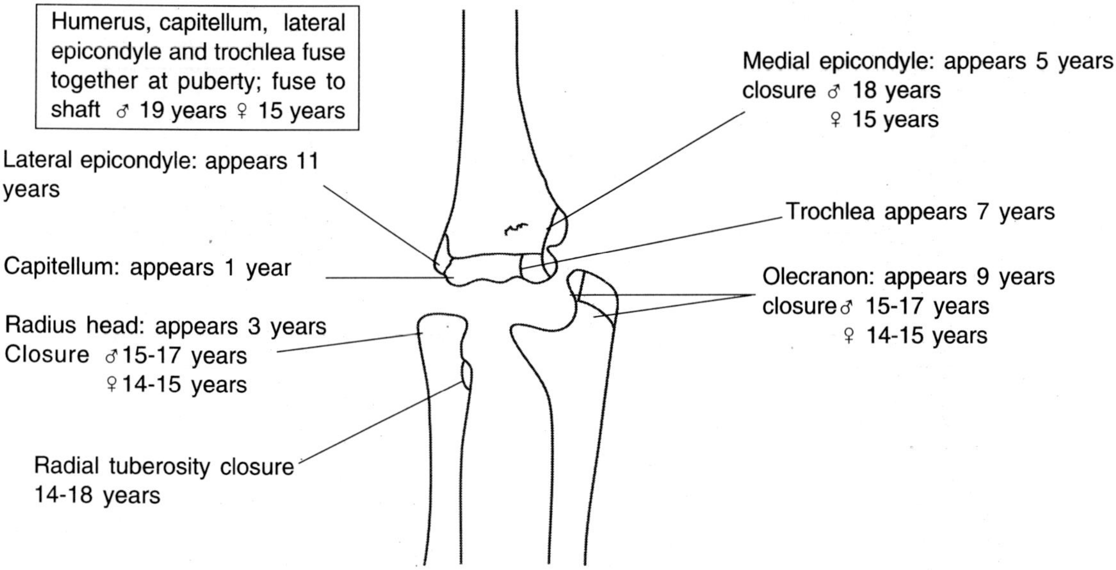

8.1A: Centres of ossification around elbow showing the age of appearance and closure

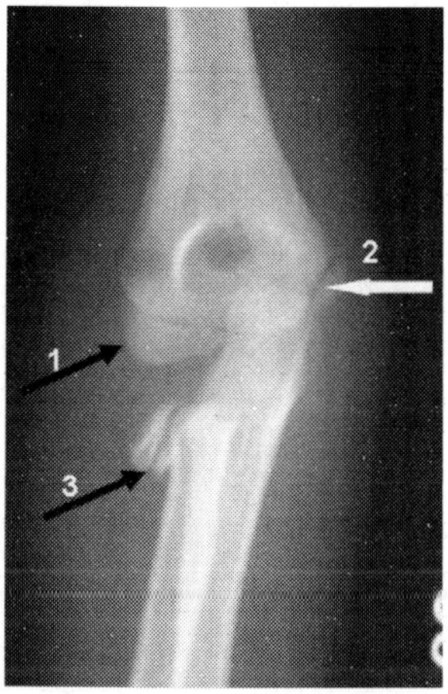

Fig. 8.1B: X-ray showing some of the centres of ossification around elbow. Arrow 1: Capitellum, Arrow 2: Medial epidcondyle; Arrow 3: Radial head (note the fracture of radial neck). As trochlear centre of ossification is not seen, the age of this child is probably between 5 to 7 years

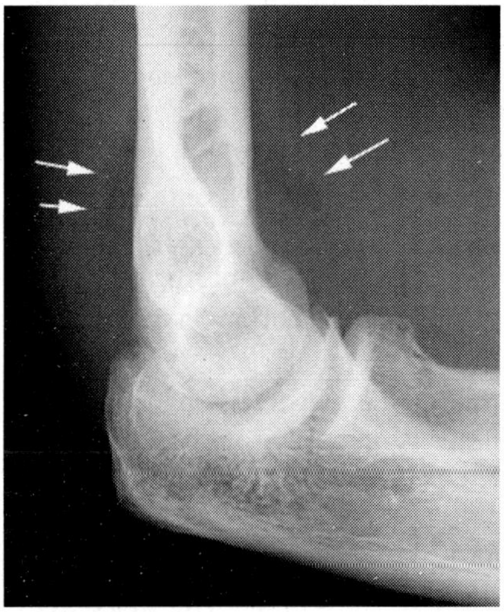

Fig. 8.2: "Fat pad sign" suggesting undisplaced fracture not visualized on X-rays

part of the elbow joint where the humerus flattens and flares. Children are particularly susceptible to this fracture between 5 to 8 years of age because (a) remodelling is occurring in this area and the bone is mainly cancellous; and, (b) hypermobile joint capsule allows the elbow to hyperextend during a fall.

Mechanism of Injury and Types

Supracondylar fractures of the humerus are of two types:

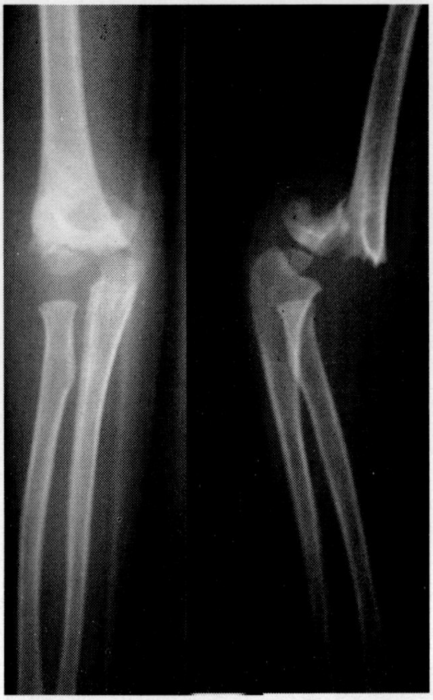

Fig. 8.3: Extension type of supracondylar fracture of humerus. Note the distal fragment is displaced backwards, upwards and medially. This is the common type

1. The Extension type (Figure 8.3) occurs when the hyperextended position drives the olecranon into the supracondylar portion of the humerus (as in fall on the out stretched hand). The distal fragment typically displaces backwards, upwards and sidewards. This type is seen in the majority of cases (~95%).
2. The flexion type (Fig. 8.4) occurs by fall on the point of a flexed elbow. The distal fragment displaces forwards, upwards and sidewards. It is uncommon pattern and is seen only in 5% cases.

Clinical Features

A child with supracondylar fracture presents with marked pain and swelling of the elbow. There is obvious deformity if the fracture is significantly displaced. However, the normal 3 bony point relationship of the olecranon, medial and lateral

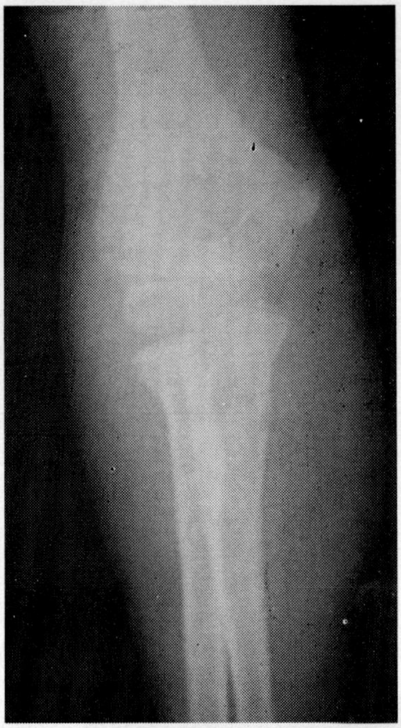

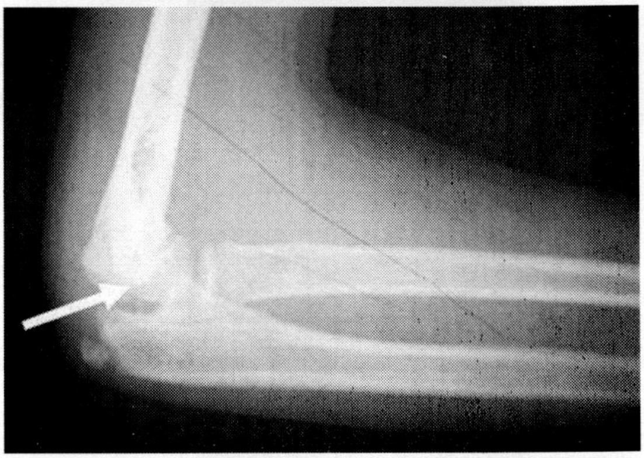

Fig. 8.4: Flexion type of supracondylar fracture. Note that the distal fragment is displaced forward (Arrow) here (c.f. the backward displacement in extension type)

condyles is maintained. Crepitus with range of motion and gross instability may be present, but it is better not to elicit these signs to avoid neurovascular injury.

A careful neurovascular evaluation is essential because the sharp fractured end of the proximal fragment may impale the brachial artery, median nerve or radial nerve.

If the patient presents late, with marked swelling, or has had massage, high index of suspicion should exist for the possibility of compartment syndrome. The signs of increasing pressure in the forearm compartments include unrelenting pain, severe swelling, pain on passive stretching of fingers and paraesthesiae. The first sign of a compartment syndrome is deranged two point discrimination.

X-rays

An AP and a lateral view focussing on the distal humerus is usually adequate. Displaced supracondylar fractures are well visualized on the lateral view.

Treatment

Undisplaced or minimally displaced fractures are treated non operatively in an above elbow POP slab in 90° flexion and forearm in neutral position for 3 weeks. After this period, the slab is removed and range of motion exercises are started.

Displaced fractures must be reduced as early as possible under general anaesthesia. Reduction maneuver involves traction in 10–15° flexion at elbow with an assistant providing the counter traction. After 3–5 minutes of traction, the sideward displacements are corrected and elbow gently flexed with pressure applied behind the distal fragment to correct the posterior tilt.

At this stage, pulse is felt. If pulse is palpable, the limb is immobilised in above elbow POP slab for 6 weeks or percutaneous pinning with K wires may be done (Fig. 8.5A, B). Flexion at the elbow above 90° is needed to stabilize the reduction as in this position triceps gets stretched and acts as an INTERNAL SPLINT.

Flexion of the elbow, in the presence of swelling around elbow, however, may compress the brachial artery thus compromising the circulation. Therefore, radial pulse must always be felt after reducing the fracture and if absent, flexion at the elbow should be reduced till the pulse returns. If it is diffcult to reduce or maintain reduction without loss of pulse, operative fixation of the fracture should be undertaken.

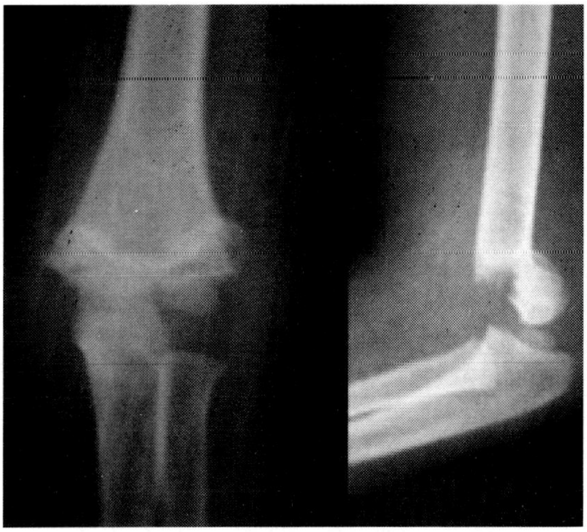

Fig. 8.5A: Extension type of supracondylar fracture of humerus

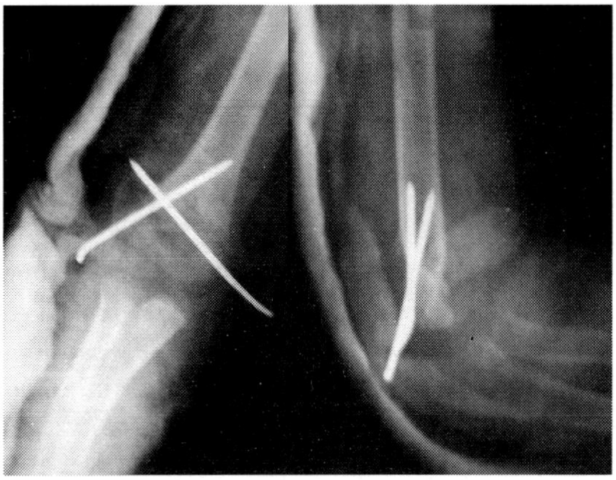

Fig. 8.5B: Fracture treated by closed reduction and percutaneous pinning using crossed K wires

Operative treatment is indicated for displaced fractures with gross swelling, vascular injury and open fractures. Most displaced fractures can be reduced by closed methods and percutaneous pinning may be done.

However, if closed reduction cannot be achieved in a severely swollen elbow, open reduction (using a medial approach) and internal fixation with K wires should be done.

The limb must be immobilized in an above elbow slab for 6 weeks after (open or closed) pinning.

Olecranon pin traction may be used in cases with vascular injury, open fractures, and in cases with gross swelling who cannot be taken up for surgery.

Supracondylar fracture with absent peripheral pulse is treated by urgent reduction of the fracture. If the circulation does not return, the brachial artery must be explored at the elbow. If the artery is lacerated it should be repaired. If it is in spasm, local papaverine application or the stripping of adventitia may relieve the spasm. If these maneuvers fail to relieve the spasm, it is probably due to the intimal tear which is treated by opening the artery, excision of the intimal tear and a vein patch if necessary.

Complications

Complications of the supracondylar fracture of the humerus can be immediate, early, delayed or late. Immediate complications include injury to brachial artery, radial nerve (most common), median or ulnar nerve.

Early complications include Volkmann ischemia which is a compartment syndrome. It is caused most commonly by tight bandage. Treatment includes immediate removal, down to skin, of all splints and dressings. If no improvement occurs, immediate fasciotomy is done for the forearm compartments on the volar aspect from the cubital fossa to the carpal tunnel. Wound is left open and covered after 4-5 days by secondary suturing or split thickness skin grafting.

Delayed complications include Volkmann's ischemic contracture (VIC) and myositis Ossificans. VIC is the aftermath of the muscle necrosis caused by the compartment syndrome. The necrotic muscles in the flexor compartment are replaced by scar tissue which contracts pulling the fingers and the wrist into flexion.

Volkmann's sign (passive extension of the fingers is possible with wrist in flexion but not with wrist in extension) is positive. It is a disabling condition and needs reconstructive surgery.

Myositis ossificans can occur after any injury around elbow and leads to stiffness.

Late complications include malunion with cubitus varus (GUNSTOCK DEFORMITY) (Fig. 8.6), which is cosmetically disabling, and stiffness. A cosmetically objectionable deformity needs correction by the supracondylar osteotomy.

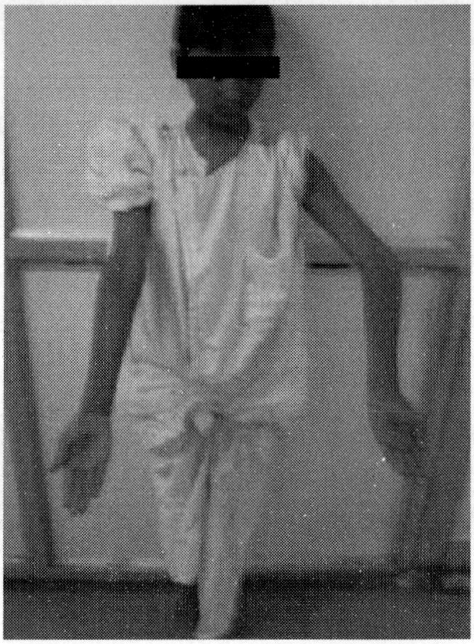

Fig. 8.6: Gunstock (cubitus varus) deformity left elbow due to malunited supracondylar fracture of humerus

Fracture of the Lateral Condyle of Humerus

Fractures of the lateral condyle of the humerus occur mainly in children. This injury represents injury to the growth plate and can produce growth disturbances and deformities at the distal humerus (Fig. 5.14). Injury to lateral condyle is commonest around the age of 6 years. Lateral condyle fracture gives rise to less satisfactory results compared to the supracondylar fractures of the humerus since (a) the fracture involves the joint, (b) there is a high incidence of growth disturbances, and, (c) the diagnosis is often missed.

Mechanisms of Injury and Types

Fractures of the lateral condyle are caused by fall leading to adduction (varus) and hyperextension force on the extended elbow. The wrist extensors attached to the lateral condyle avulse a large fragment. There are two types of lateral condyle fractures as shown in figure. Fortunately type II (which is Salter-Harris type II and less likely to lead to growth disturbance) is more common.

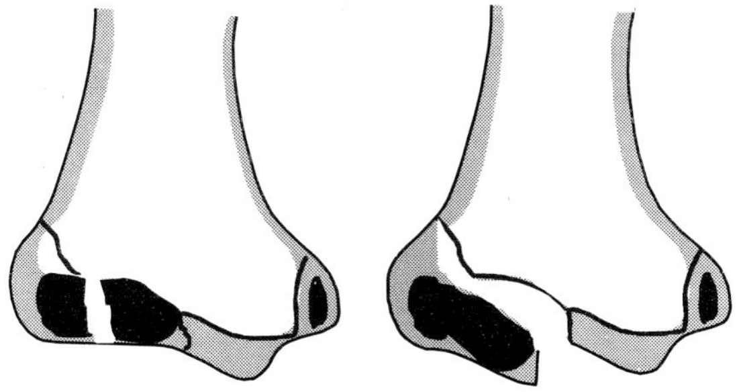

Fig. 8.7: Types of fracture of lateral condyle of humerus

Clinical Features

Unlike the supracondylar fracture of the humerus, the patient presents with less obvious findings and the diagnosis may be missed in subtle cases. Patient presents with swelling (which is often mild and most prominent over the lateral aspect of distal humerus), limited ROM, and tenderness over the injured condyle. Crepitation with motion (especially with pronation-supination) is often present.

X-rays

Two views-AP and lateral of the elbow are adequate to diagnose lateral condyle fracture (Fig. 8.8). Since the capitellar epiphysis is largely cartilaginous, the bony fragment looks much smaller on the X-rays compared to its real size. The fragment is displaced as well as frequently rotated due to the pull of attached extensors.

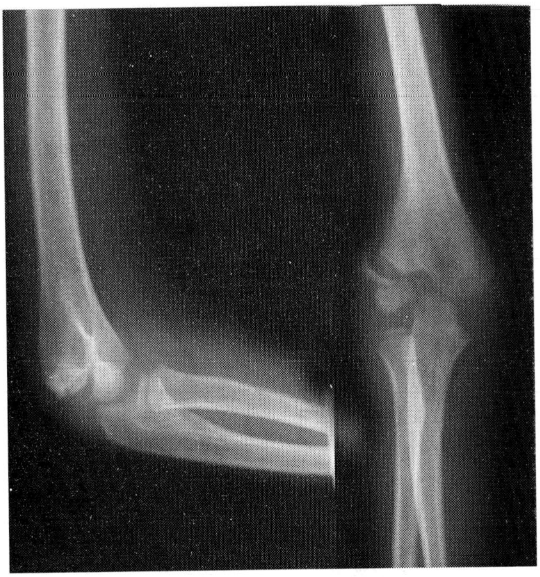

Fig. 8.8: Fracture lateral condyle of humerus

Treatment

Undisplaced or minimally displaced (< 2 mm) fracture can be treated in the above elbow POP cast with elbow flexed 90°, forearm in neutral rotation and wrist slightly extended for 3 to 4 weeks. Repeat X-rays should be taken every 3-5 days for the first 2 weeks to ensure that the fracture has not displaced. Range of motion exercises are started after removal of plaster.

Open reduction is required for displaced fracture. After reduction, the fracture is fixed by passing two smooth Kirschner wires (Fig. 8.9). (Note: Passage of smooth wires does not result in growth disturbance). Post operatively, the elbow is immobilised in long-arm cast at 90° with the forearm in neutral rotation. Cast is kept for 6–8 weeks followed by pin removal and active range of motion exercises.

Complications

1. Delayed or non union occurs due to poor vascularity of lateral condylar fragment and pull of extensors. It may result in cubitus valgus leading to tardy ulnar nerve palsy (vide infera).

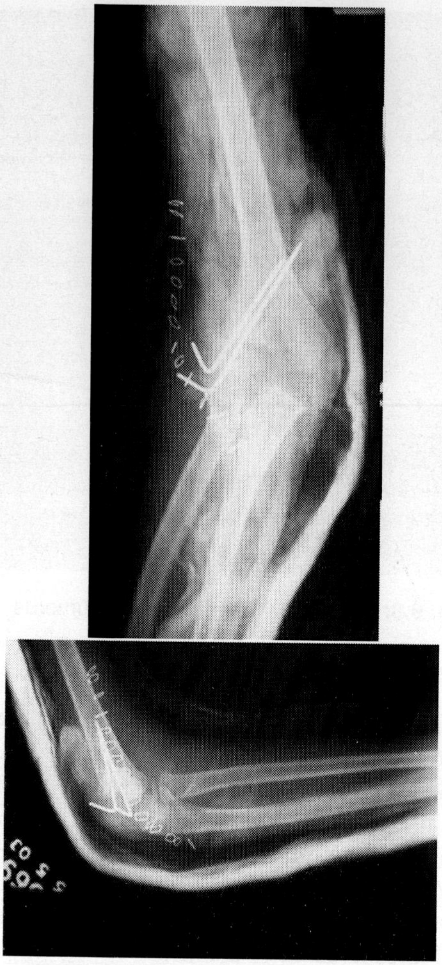

Fig. 8.9: Lateral condyle fracture of humerus treated by open reduction and K wire pinning

Treatment ranges from neglect (non union or malunion) to corrective osteotomy at supra-condylar level (no attempt is made to achieve union at fracture for nonunion).

2. Angular deformities: cubitus valgus more commonly than varus due to the growth arrest of lateral physis.
3. Tardy ulnar nerve palsy may occur more than 10–15 years after injury due to friction as the deformed elbow with cubitus valgus is moved in flexion-extension. The treatment comprises of anterior transposition of the ulnar nerve.
4. Avascular necrosis: of the fragment may occur especially in cases of late surgery and may lead to "fish-tail" deformity.
5. Myositis ossificans may occur rarely.

Fracture of Medial Epicondyle

Medial epicondyle is a traction apophysis for the medial collateral ligament and wrist flexors and does not contribute to humeral length. Fractures of the medial epicondyle occur mainly between 9 to 12 years of age and are often associated with fracture of the proximal radius, olecranon and coronoid or with dislocation of the elbow.

Mechanism of Injury

"Pull-off" by the valgus force (as in fall on outstretched hand) is common but direct trauma to the posterior or postero lateral aspect of medial epicondyle may sometimes be responsible. If the injury causes the elbow joint to open up on medial side, the fragment may be pulled into the joint space.

Clinical Features

Patient presents with pain, swelling and tenderness over the medial aspect of the joint. Resisted wrist flexion (due to pull of wrist flexors on the fractured fragment) aggravates the symptoms. Ulnar nerve may be injured during trauma or from swelling over medial aspect of elbow and a careful neuro-vascular examination should be performed in all cases. ROM is decreased secondary to pain. An entrapped fragment in the joint causes mechanical block to range of motion.

X-rays

Anteroposterior and lateral X-ray of the elbow should be taken (Fig. 8.10). The fracture is often missed and radiographs of the two elbows should be compared carefully to diagnose the presence or the absence of the fracture. Complete absence of the apophysis on standard elbow views should lead to suspicion of fracture or incarceration of the

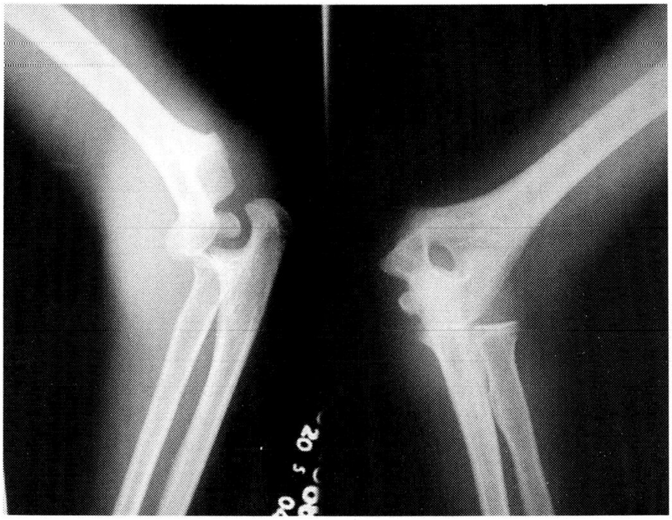

Fig. 8.10: AP and lateral view of displaced medial epicondyle fracture of humerus. Incarceration of fragment into the joint is suggested on X-rays by visualization of the fragment at the level of joint line. The patient also had ulnar nerve injury

fragment within the joint as in that case it may be obscured by distal humerus. Visualization of the fracture fragment at the level of the joint line on X-rays suggests incarceration of the fragment in the joint.

Treatment

Most fractures can be treated non operatively with good results. An above elbow POP slab with elbow and wrist flexed and the forearm pronated is applied for 10–14 days and then discontinued and active motion exercises are begun. Fracture usually joins with fibrous tissue but good or excellent functional results are seen in nearly 96% cases. Operative treatment is indicated in case of an irreducible and incarcerated fragment within the elbow joint. During surgery, ulnar nerve is identified and retracted, fragment is delivered from the joint, reduced and fixed with Kirschner wires or a screw. Following surgery, above elbow POP slab is given for 10–14 days followed by ROM exercises.

Complications

1. Ulnar nerve palsy: Stretching of the nerve may occur due to the valgus strain that causes fracture. Cases associated with entrapped fragment may have up to 50% incidence of ulnar nerve dysfunction.
2. Non union: may occur in up to 60% cases with significant displacement but is hardly a functional problem.
3. Loss of extension may occur in almost 20% cases.
4. Myositis ossificans is rare and occurs if fracture is repeatedly and vigorously manipulated.

Radial Head and Neck Fracture

Radial head and neck fractures both can occur in adults but radial head fractures are more common. However, in children radial head fractures are rare and neck fractures relatively more common. These injuries occur most commonly due to fall on the outstretched hand. A valgus force at elbow can also fracture radial head. Elbow dislocations may be associated with radial head or neck fractures.

Clinical Features

Patient has diffuse swelling over lateral elbow and limitation of ROM, especially forearm rotations and elbow extension. Direct, gentle thumb pressure over the radial head at posterolateral elbow elicits acute discomfort, especially with gentle passive pronation and supination. Crepitus may sometimes be elicited by this maneuver.

X-rays: Standard AP and lateral views of elbow can be supplemented by "Radial head view" which is an oblique X-ray with elbow at 90° flexion (Fig. 8.11). Radial head fractures may be missed often and X-rays may have to be taken in different rotations of forearm (Fig. 8.12).

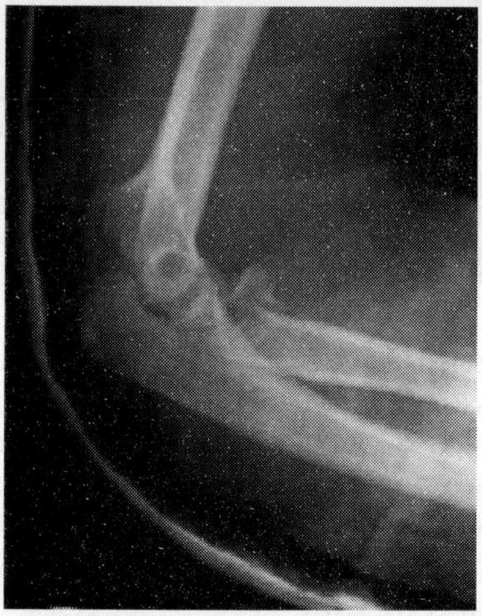

Fig. 8.11: Radial head fracture. Note the displacement of fragment

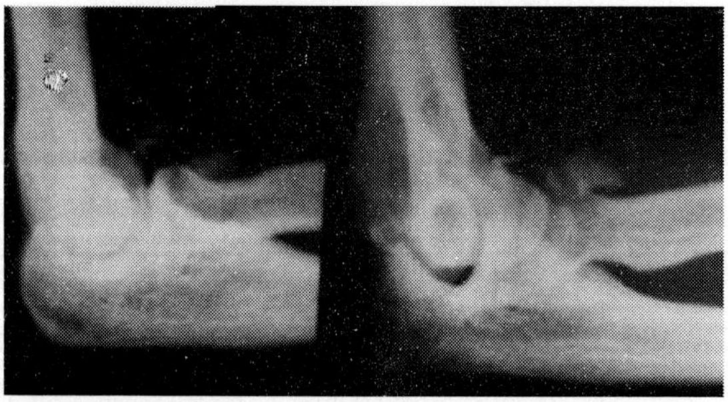

Fig. 8.12: Importance of view in different rotations for radial head fracture. The view on the left did not reveal the fracture which is seen when X-ray was taken in a different rotation

Note should be made of the number of fragments and their displacement. Common associated fractures include the olecranon, coronoid and medial epicondyle. Radial neck fractures are typically mildly or moderately impacted (Fig. 8.13).

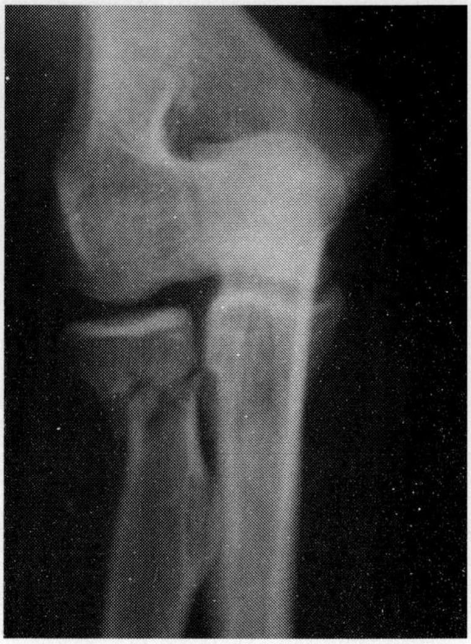

Fig. 8.13: Radial neck fracture. These fractures are often impacted or minimally displaced.

Treatment is non operative for undisplaced fractures. A sling is given for the first 5-7 days till pain is bearable and then the elbow is mobilized.

Single large displaced fragment of radial head which is more than 1/3rd of head, displaced 3 mm or more or angulated more than 30 degrees is fixed (commonly with screws). Comminuted radial head fractures are treated by excision of the radial head.

Radial neck fractures angulated more than 30° are treated by closed reduction to reduce displacement. Failure to achieve closed reduction is treated with open reduction with or without internal fixation. Excision of radial head is never done in children as it leads to instability at elbow and disruption of radio ulnar articulations.

Complications

1. Stiffness: The range of pronation, supination, extension and flexion is reduced in that order.
2. Radioulnar synostosis is the most serious complication which can occur following manipulations and surgery. Rotations are completely absent and osteotomy is required to restore function.
3. Myositis ossificans may occur.

4. Osteoarthritis occurs if the articular incongruity persists following treatment.

Intercondylar Fractures of Humerus

Intercondylar fractures of humerus are caused by a direct blow to the elbow driving the olecranon into distal humerus disrupting condyles. Injury is common in adults and rare in children. The fractures are displaced in T or Y fashion (Fig. 8.14). Patient presents with swelling with or without bruising around elbow. Forearm appears shortened in cases where proximal migration of ulna occurs following fracture. Diagnosis is obvious on routine X-rays (AP and lateral). Treatment for undisplaced fracture is conservative in POP slab for 8-10 weeks and for displaced fractures, open reduction and internal fixation is done using plates and screws followed by immediate ROM exercises.

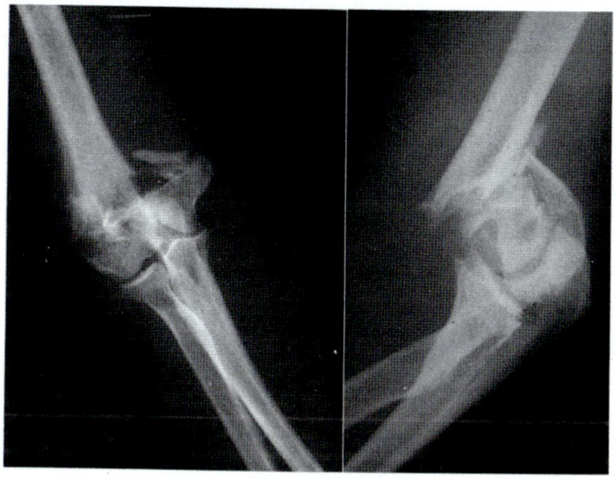

Fig. 8.14: Comminuted T shaped intercondylar fracture of distal humerus

Complications include stiffness of elbow, nonunion or malunion and osteoarthritis of elbow.

Dislocation of Elbow

Dislocation of elbow is third in frequency after shoulder and finger joints. These dislocations occur in young active population and are often associated with sports injuries. There is a high incidence of associated fractures including those of the medial epicondyle, coronoid and radial head and neck.

Mechanism and Types

Elbow dislocation occurs most commonly due to fall on outstretched hand with hyperextension at elbow.

Elbow dislocations are classified according to the position of the ulna relative to the humerus after injury. Posterior dislocations are more common and most of these are posterolateral (> 90%). Other types are anterior, lateral, medial and divergent (rare). Anterior dislocation cannot occur without fracture of the olecranon.

Clinical Features

Dislocation of elbow is hard to miss. Patient presents with swelling, deformity and inability to move elbow. Triceps is taut and there is reversal of 3 bony point relationship on the posterior aspect of the elbow (Fig. 8.15). A careful neurovascular examination must be performed immediately (before radiographs) and following any manipulation or reduction. Brachial artery injury should be suspected in cases with massive antecubital swelling and poor distal perfusion. After reduction if perfusion is not restored patient should be taken

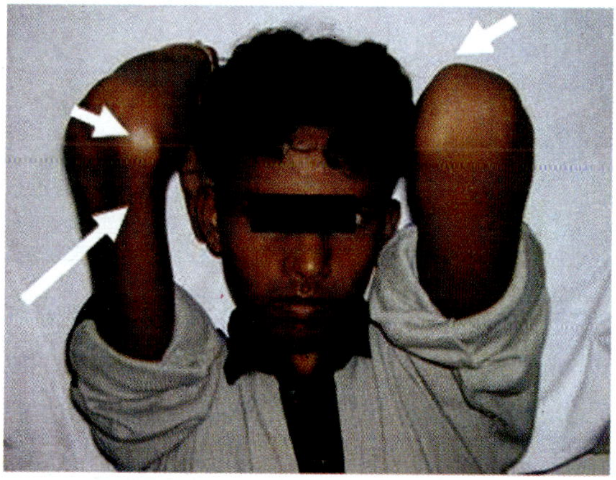

Fig. 8.15: Posterior dislocation of right elbow: Clinical photograph. Note that the triceps is taut (long arrow) and the tip of olecranon on the dislocated side has moved proximally compared to the normal (left) side (Small arrow) demonstrating the reversal of 3 bony point relationship

up for angiography followed by arterial reconstruction. Note that radial pulse may be present with brachial artery compromise as a result of collateral circulation. Compartment syndrome should be looked for and diagnosed early if present.

X-Rays

Standard AP and lateral X-ray are taken to confirm the presence and the direction of the dislocation (Fig. 8.16) as well as to evaluate for associated fractures about the elbow.

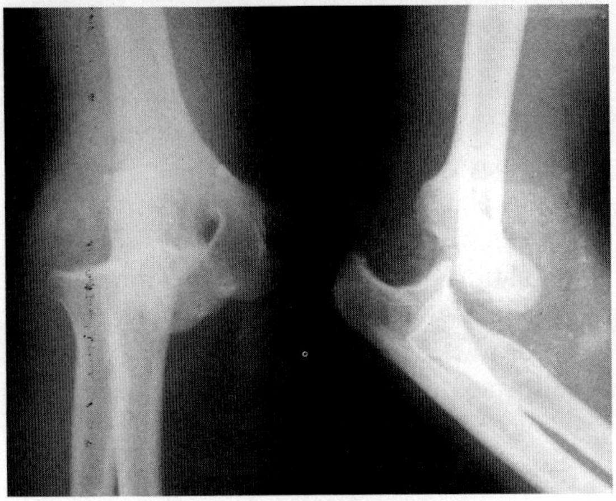

Fig. 8.16: Posterolateral dislocation of (R) elbow joint

Treatment

Acute posterior dislocation is managed initially with closed reduction under sedation and analgesia or GA. Reduction is performed with elbow flexed while distal traction is applied in line with forearm. Following reduction neurovascular status is reassessed followed by the evaluation of range of motion with stability. Radiographs are taken and POP slab applied in 90° flexion at elbow. Early, gentle ROM exercises are started at 3 weeks.

Complications

1. Neurovascular compromise: Brachial artery is most commonly disrupted due to injury. Median, ulnar and radial nerves are involved in decreasing frequency. Spontaneous recovery of nerve function usually occurs following closed injury.
2. Compartment syndrome.
3. Instability/Redislocation: can occur in the presence of associated coronoid process fracture and radial head fracture (Terrible triad of elbow).
4. Stiffness of elbow, especially loss of extension.
5. Myositis ossificans.

Fracture of Olecranon

Incidence of fracture of olecranon has two peaks; first occurs in young people due to high energy trauma and the second in older age due to falls. A fracture of olecranon with displacement represent a functional disruption of the triceps mechanism, resulting in loss of active extension of the elbow (This is analogous to displaced fracture of patella representing a functional disruption of the quadriceps mechanism, leading to loss of active extension at the knee).

Mechanism and Types

Olecranon may be fractured by (a) direct injury due to fall on the point of elbow or direct trauma to elbow. This leads to comminuted fracture; (b) Indirect injury when a fall on the out stretched hand accompanied by a strong sudden contraction of the triceps typically leads to a transverse or oblique fracture.

The olecranon fracture can be undisplaced or displaced, it can be oblique and transverse (due to indirect injury) or comminuted (direct trauma); and it may be isolated or a part of fracture-dislocation of the elbow.

Clinical Features

Patient presents with swelling around elbow and the upper extremity supported by the opposite hand. Abrasions over elbow or hand may suggest the mechanism. Palpation may reveal a palpable defect or gap at the fracture site. Patient is unable to extend the elbow actively against gravity indicating discontinuity of the triceps mechanism. A careful neurological examination should be performed to rule out associated ulnar nerve injury.

X-Rays

Standard AP and lateral radiographs are sufficient (Fig. 8.17) and give information about extent of fracture, displacement, comminution, and the presence or absence of other injuries (such as elbow dislocation or radial head fracture).

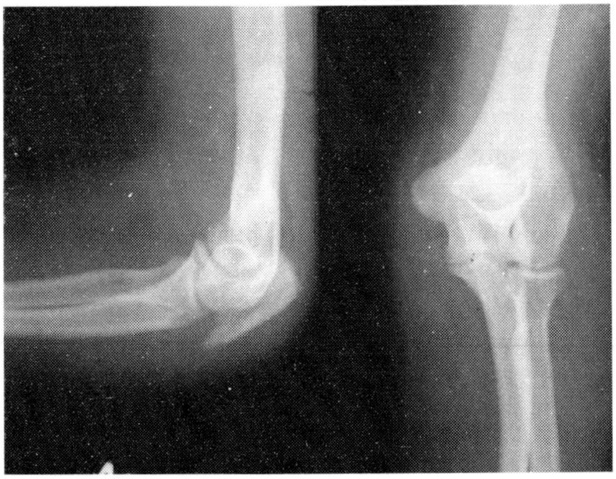

Fig. 8.17: Fracture of the olecranon

Treatment

Undisplaced fractures are treated in long arm cast in 45-90° flexion for 3 weeks followed by gentle ROM exercises. Follow up check X-rays are performed after 1 week to rule out redisplacement.

Displaced fractures (> 2 mm; suggesting disruption of triceps mechanism) are treated by open reduction and internal fixation using tension band wiring, intramedullary screw fixation or plate and screw fixation (Fig. 8.18). Extensively comminuted fractures can be treated by excision of olecranon and reattachment of triceps tendon. Post operatively, elbow is immobilised in a posterior slab in 45-90° flexion.

Complications

1. Stiffness of the elbow.

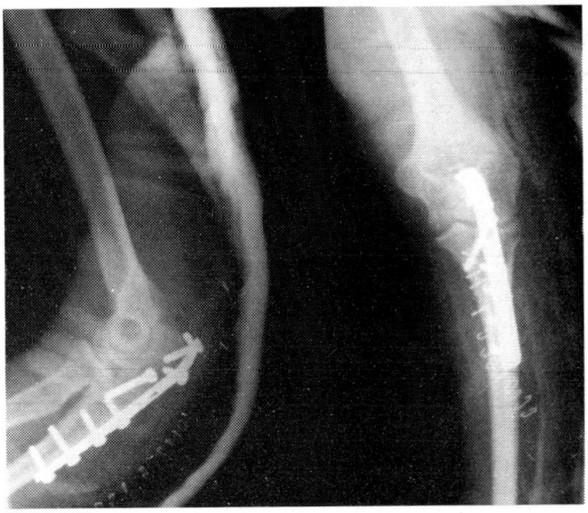

Fig. 8.18: Fracture olecranon treated by plate and screws

2. Post traumatic arthritis (especially with > 2 mm step in articular surface)
3. Non union
4. Weakness of extension

Radial Head Subluxation ("Pulled elbow"; Nurse maid's elbow)

Pulled elbow occurs in children around 2-3 years age (range 6 mo to 6 years). It is caused by longitudinal traction force on extended elbow in pronation. Patient presents with history of sudden longitudinal traction applied to extended upper extremity (as holding child by hand and pulling up from bed) often with audible snap. The child stops using the extremity (pseudoparalysis) and hangs it in dependent position, with elbow slightly flexed. X-rays are interpreted as normal though ultrasound has been shown to be of some help. Condition should be differentiated from septic arthritis or proximal radius fractures. Treatment consists of closed reduction which is achieved by firm supination of forearm with thumb pressure on the radial head and elbow flexion. A palpable click is felt upon reduction. Recovery of child is dramatic and the child starts reusing the hand almost immediately. Post operative immobilization or X-rays are unnecessary.

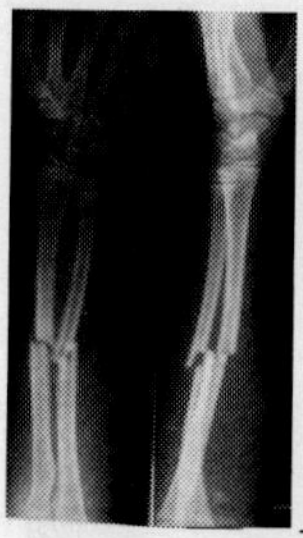

9 Injuries of the Forearm, Wrist and Hand

Forearm bones, Distal Radius, Carpal injuries, Metacarpals, Phalanges, Dislocations in Hand, Gamekeeper's thumb

Injuries of the forearm, wrist and hand are among the most common injuries encountered in the emergency. Lack of proper management of any of these injuries will lead to compromised function of the upper extremity. It is therefore, extremely important to pay careful attention to detail while treating these injuries.

INJURIES OF THE FOREARM

The radius and ulna are mechanically interconnected by the superior and inferior radio-ulnar joints and the interosseous membrane. It is therefore, difficult to break one bone without breaking or dislocating the other. The following principles should be kept in mind while treating forearm injuries:

1. If one forearm bone is fractured and displaced, and the other bone looks intact, carefully look for the dislocation of the superior or inferior radio ulnar joint.
2. A direct injury to forearm leads to transverse fractures almost at the same level; an indirect (fall on the outstretched hand) injury leads to short oblique or spiral fractures—usually at different levels.
3. The attachment of supinator/pronator muscles to different regions of the forearm bones requires that the distal fragments are appropriately positioned so that they align anatomically with proximal fragments. For example in the proximal third fractures of the both bones of the forearm, proximal fragments are supinated because of the attachment of supinator muscle on the radius. If the distal forearm is supinated, reduction will be readily achieved. Likewise for the mid third fractures, forearm is positioned mid way (mid-prone or mid supinated). In the distal third fractures, pronators are attached to proximal radius and distal forearm has to be pronated to align the fragments.
4. Normal rotation of forearm requires restoring the proper rotational alignment of forearm bones (i.e. restoring the normal anatomy of the interosseous membrane), length and the normal bow of the radius and normal superior and inferior radio-ulnar joints. Union of the forearm bones in malrotation or persistent subluxation or dislocation of the superior or inferior radio-ulnar joint will lead to loss of the forearm rotations.
5. Communicating haematomas of the two bones (due to fractures at the same level with torn interosseous membrane or due to open reduction and internal fixation of both bones through a single incision) will lead to cross union with consequent loss of all the rotations at the forearm.
6. Forearm has limited space within rigid fibro-osseous compartments. As the fractures invariably lead to swelling, a high index of suspicion should be maintained for the compartment syndrome.

Fractures of Both the Forearm Bones

Fractures of both bones of the forearm are common in both children and adults. In children they are usually greenstick or torus fractures (Chapter 1) or, if displaced, are easily reduced and maintained in plaster. In adults these fractures are often oblique and difficult to maintain in plaster and treat conservatively.

Mechanism of Injury and Types

The most common mechanism of injury is fall on the outstretched hand (indirect); sometimes it can be direct hit on the forearm.

The forearm bones may be fractured at the same level or at different levels. In either case the fracture of the respective bone is described as in upper third, mid third or the lower third. The fractures may be closed or open, displaced or undisplaced and simple or comminuted.

Clinical Features

Patient presents with signs and symptoms of fracture, including pain, swelling, deformity, abnormal mobility, crepitation and loss of hand and forearm function. Physical examination should include assessment of soft tissues, including gentle palpation for possible compartment syndrome, examination of the elbow and wrist and the evaluation of neurovascular status.

X-rays

Radiographs should include anteroposterior (AP) and lateral views of forearm as well as the elbow and wrist (Fig. 9.1).

X-rays should be evaluated for the location, configuration, comminution and displacement of the fracture fragments and the status of the neighbouring joints.

Treatment

In children these injuries are treated by closed reduction and immobilization in above elbow (axilla to metacarpal necks with elbow flexed 90° and forearm neutral) plaster for 6 weeks. Weekly check X-rays for 2 weeks are taken to rule out redisplacement of these fractures if they were initially manipulated.

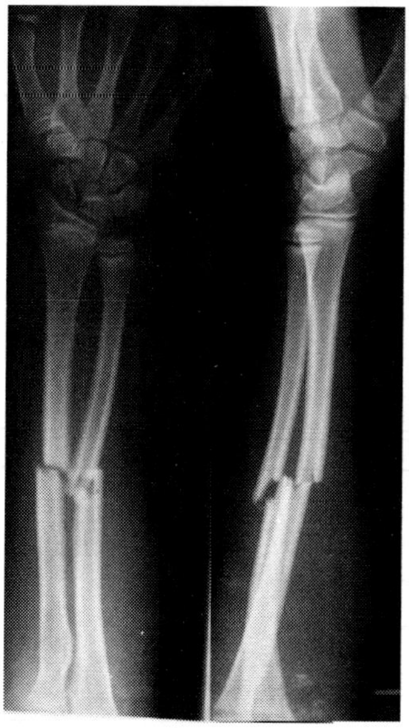

Fig. 9.1: Fracture both bones of the forearm in middle third

In adults, only undisplaced or minimally displaced (these are, however, uncommon) fractures are treated conservatively in the above elbow POP cast for 12 weeks. Displaced fractures are treated by open reduction and internal fixation using plates and screws. Sometimes, in cases such as segmental fractures or in the presence of wound over the planned incision area for plating, intramedullary nailing may be done (Fig. 9.2). Ulnar nails are introduced from the olecranon while the radial nails are introduced from distal end, either through the radial styloid or Lister's tubercle. While external plaster immobilization is often not required after the forearm bones have been rigidly fixed by plating, plaster must be applied after the intramedullary nailing which has poor control over rotation of the fragments. Fractures take about 12 weeks to heal.

Fracture of a Single Bone

Fractures of the single bone without any associated injury are uncommon. When present, these fractures are undisplaced and may be easily missed. Sometimes these may be initially displaced with dislocation of neighbouring radio-ulnar joint but have been subsequently reduced. The pain and

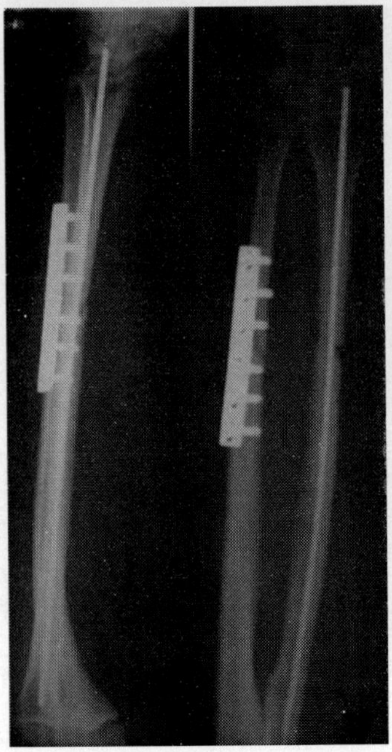

Fig. 9.2: Fractures of both bones of forearm are treated by open reduction and plates and screws fixation in adults. However, in case of wound over incision area for plating or in case of segmental fracture, one or both bones can be fixed by intra medullary (Talwalkar) nail

tenderness over the concerned radio-ulnar joint may suggest that the joint was injured initially.

a. Isolated undisplaced fracture of radius is treated in an above elbow POP cast for 6 weeks followed by below elbow cast till the fracture is healed. A fracture of radius in adult which is displaced (>10° angulation and >50% shaft displacement) is treated by open reduction and internal fixation using plate and screws.
b. An isolated fracture of ulnar shaft (Night Stick or Parry fracture) (Fig. 9.3) is caused when one is trying to ward off or parry away an attack by sticks. The usually undisplaced fracture is treated in an above elbow cast. Displaced ulnar fractures (>10° angulated and >50% shaft displacement) are treated by open reduction and plate and screws fixation. Since there are sparse soft tissue attachments over the distal ulna, the delayed union and non union are common.

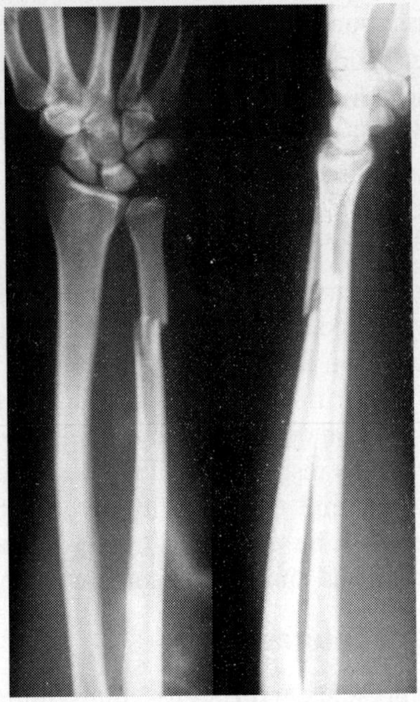

Fig. 9.3: Isolated minimally displaced ulna fracture ("Night stick injury"). These fractures are usually treated conservatively

Fracture-Dislocations

Two Italians described the principle that the two-bone unit of radius and ulna does not allow one bone to fracture and shorten without breaking or dislocating the other bone. The key to success in treating these cases is to restore the length of shortened bone. Only then the associated dislocation can be reduced.

a. Monteggia's fracture is the fracture of proximal ulna with dislocation of the radial head (Fig. 9.4A). It is important not to miss radial head dislocation. A displaced radial head can injure posterior interosseous nerve in about 20% cases. The treatment of Monteggia's fracture in children is closed reduction and plaster immobilisation. The common anterior dislocation of the radial head requires flexing elbow above 90° to reduce radial head and maintain reduction. In adults open reduction and internal fixation of the ulna fracture is performed followed by reduction of the radial head (often it reduces spontaneously with reduction of the ulna

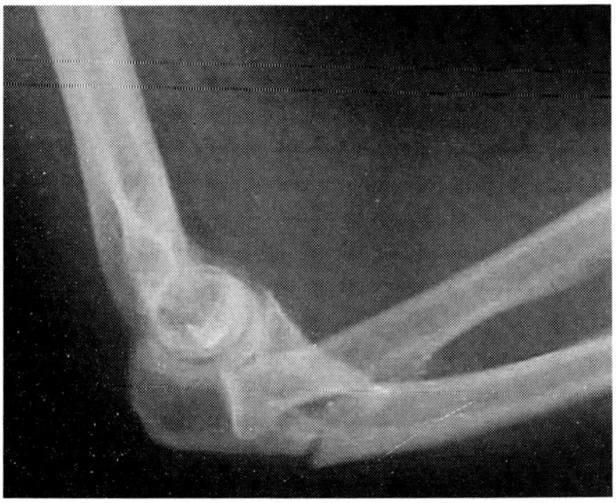

Fig. 9.4A: Monteggia fracture dislocation. There is posterior angulation of ulna fracture with posterior dislocation of radial head.

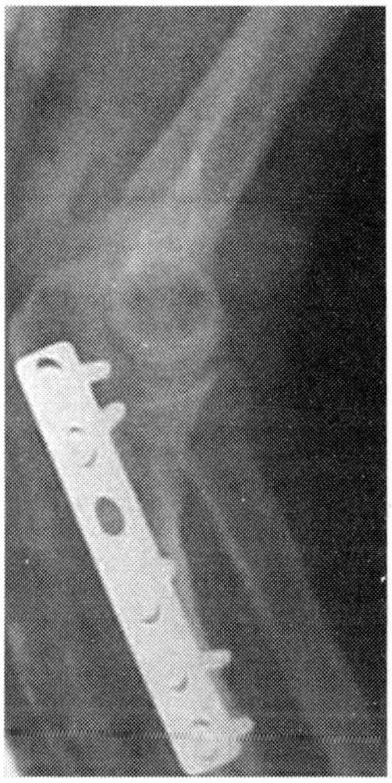

Fig. 9.4B: Montegia fracture dislocation in adult treated by plating. Note that the radial head is now reduced.

fracture) and immobilisation of elbow in above 90° flexion (Fig. 9.4B). Immobilization is continued for 6 weeks.

b. Galeazzi's fracture (or Piedmont fracture) is the fracture of the distal radial diaphysis (usually at the junction of the middle and the distal thirds) with associated disruption of the distal radio-ulnar joint (Fig. 9.5A). Galeazzi fractures are nearly three times as common as Monteggia fractures. It is also called the **fracture of necessity** as it requires reduction and internal fixation for achieving a good result.

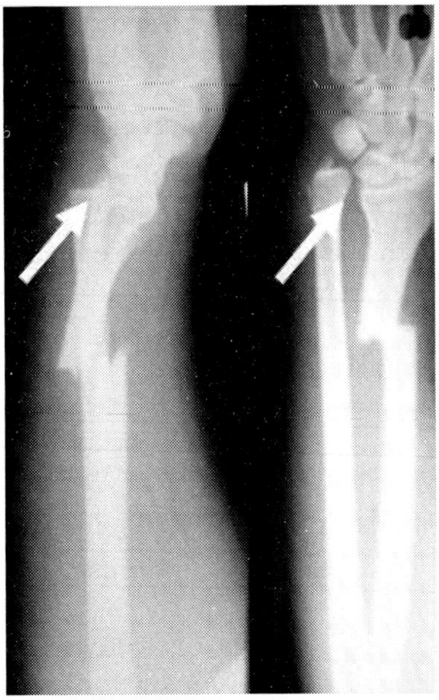

Fig. 9.5A: Galeazzi fracture dislocation. Note the disruption of inferior radioulnar joint (arrow)

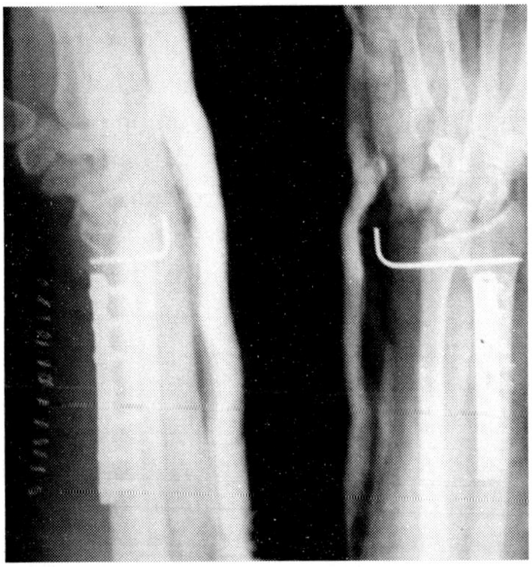

Fig. 9.5B: Galeazzi fracture treated by open reduction and plating of radius fracture. Inferior radioulnar joint was unstable in this case and had to be fixed with K-wire.

The Galeazzi fracture is treated by open reduction and internal fixation of the radius fracture using plate and screws (Fig. 9.5B). The distal radioulnar joint can usually be reduced in supination and then the above elbow plaster is applied with elbow in 90° flexion and forearm in supination for 6 weeks.

c. *Essex Lopresti injury* is a fracture of the radial head with disruption of the interosseous membrane leading to proximal migration of radius and disruption of the inferior radioulnar joint. Excision of the radial head is contraindicated in these cases to avoid proximal migration of the radius and further disruption of the distal radioulnar joint.

Complications of Forearm Fractures

1. Compartment syndrome: Urgent fasciotomy should be done if the compartment syndrome is diagnosed.
2. Nerve injury: Posterior interosseous nerve is injured in Monteggia's fracture dislocations. Nerve injury may also occur due to missile projectile injuries.
3. Non union is common in open fractures, severely comminuted fractures, fractures with bone loss or in cases with inadequate fixation (Fig. 9.6). Treatment of non union of ulna and radius is plate and screw fixation with autogenous bone grafts taken from the iliac crest.
4. Malunion results from poor initial reduction or inadequate skeletal stabilization. Corrective osteotomy with plating and bone grafting may be required if the malunion is interfering with function. Corrective osteotomy of malunited ulna is mandatory in neglected/maltreated Monteggia fracture without which the radial head remains dislocated. In children attempt is made to relocate radial head if child presents within 3 months of injury; in adults the radial head is excised.
5. Post traumatic radioulnar synostosis (Cross Union) is uncommon (3 to 9% cases) yet devastating complication. It can occur following Monteggia fracture, high energy fractures with comminution or when both bones are fixed through a single incision. Loss of rotation occurs. Excision of synostosis can be undertaken one year after injury but the results are not encouraging.
6. Infection occurs following open reduction and internal fixation or open fractures. It is treated by repeated surgical debridement, wound culture and appropriate antibiotics. External fixation may be required with wound left open if necessary in case of massive infections.

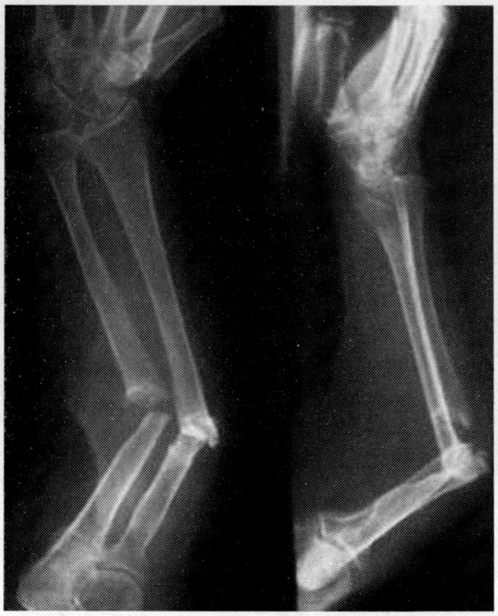

Fig. 9.6: Non union both bones of the forearm with lateral and dorsal angulation. This patient was not treated adequately with plaster (Inadequate immobilization) and the fracture went to non union

INJURIES AROUND THE WRIST

Distal Radius Fractures

Distal radius fractures are among the most common fractures of the upper extremity (17%). They have bimodal distribution, the more commonly affected elderly population sustains this fracture due to osteoporosis while the younger patients sustain this fracture due to high-energy trauma. The following principles must be kept in mind while treating distal radius fractures:

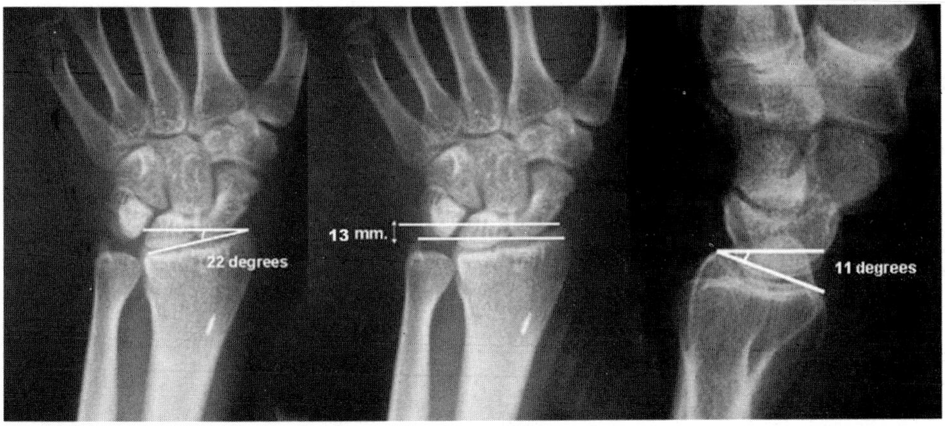

Fig. 9.7: Normal radio graphic relationships of wrist joint (Left) Ulnar tilt; (Middle) Radial length; (Right) Volar tilt

1. Distal radius is mainly composed of cancellous bone. Fractures at the cortico-cancellous junction lead to impaction of soft distal bone in proximal shaft fragment leading to shortening of radius.
2. Following a fracture, distal radius cannot shorten without disruption of inferior radioulnar joint, fracture of the ulnar styloid process or the tear of the triangular fibro cartilage. The triangular cartilage attaches to the base of ulnar styloid and carpus on ulnar side and radius on the other side.
3. Normally tip of radial styloid is 13 mm (average; range 8-18 mm) distal to the tip of ulnar styloid and this must be restored after fracture treatment along with the restoration of inclination of the distal radius fragment.

5. The normal radiographic relationships in the wrist joint are (Fig. 9.7):
   - Ulnar tilt : average 22 degrees
   - Volar tilt : average 11 degrees
   - Radial length : average 13 mm
5. Stiffness (especially fingers and shoulder) is the most common complication following these fractures and patient should be encouraged to move his fingers, elbow and shoulder at all times.

Mechanism of Injury and Types

The most common mechanism of injury is fall on the out stretched hand, with the wrist in dorsiflexion. This may happen following a low energy impact in an elderly osteoporotic patient. In younger patients these fractures occur following high energy impact as in falls from height, motor vehicle accidents or athletic injuries.

The distal radius fractures can be classified into various types and these types are often identified by eponyms:

1. *Colles' fracture (Fig. 9.8):* A fracture of distal radius at the cortico-cancellous junction (within 1 inch of articular surface; extra-articular) with

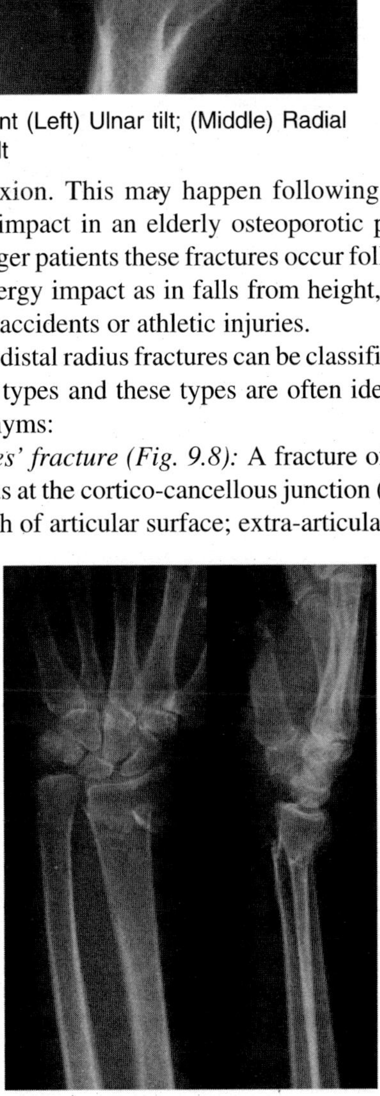

Fig. 9.8: Colles' fracture. Note the typical displacements

typical, 6 displacements namely, Dorsal tilt, Dorsal displacement, Lateral tilt, Lateral displacement, impaction and supination. The classical "Dinner fok" deformity is typical of this fracture (Fig. 9.9).

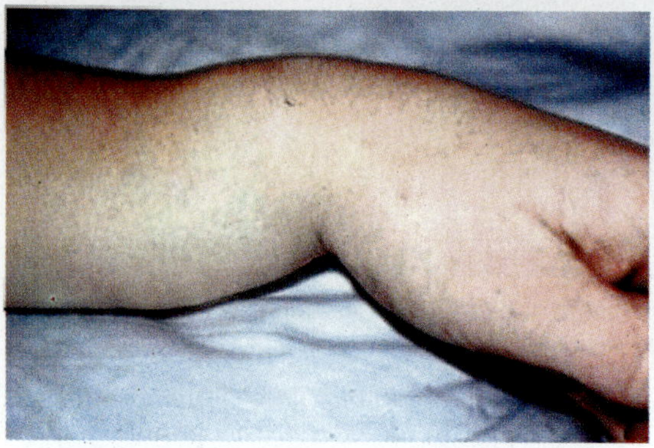

Fig. 9.9: Dinner fork deformity resulting from malunion of Colles' fracture

2. *Smith's fracture (Fig. 9.10):* is a "reverse Colles" fracture with opposite (volar) displacement. The deformity is often described as "Garden spade" deformity.

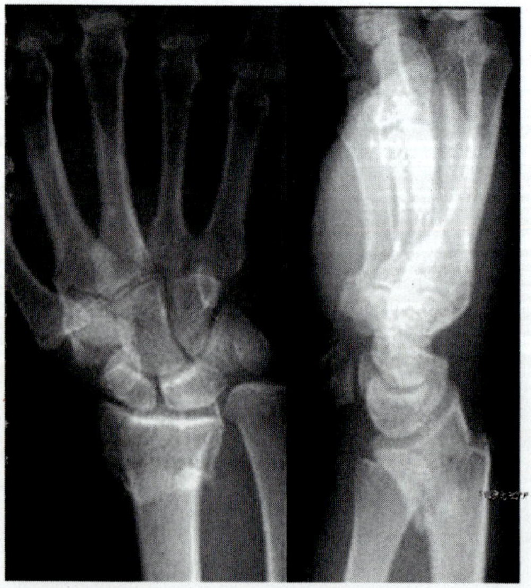

Fig. 9.10: Smith's fracture

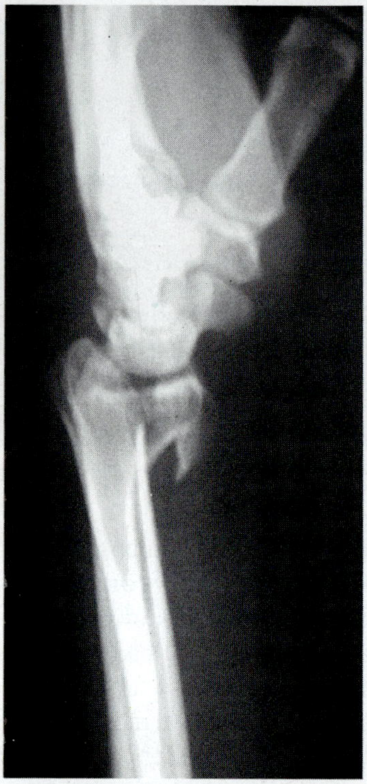

Fig. 9.11: Volar Barton fracture. Note the anterior subluxation of the carpus

3. *Barton's fractures (Fig. 9.11):* Are intra articular fractures of distal radius with instability of carpus (fracture—dislocation of wrist)—can be dorsal or volar lip fractures of radius with carpal subluxation.
4. *Chauffeur's Fracture:* Fracture of radial styloid.
5. *Die punch (Lunate load):* Intra articular depression fracture of lunate fossa of the articular surface of the distal radius.

Colles' Fracture

This constitutes more than 90% of distal radius fractures. Colles' fracture was described by Abraham Colles in 1814. The characteristic deformity caused by this fracture (caused by fall on the outstretched hand in an elderly osteoporotic person, usually postmenopausal woman), is "dinner fork" deformity because the wrist and hand look in profile like a fork turned tines down.

Clinical Features

Patient presents with gross deformity of the wrist (marked dorsal prominence caused by dorsal displacement of distal fragment) with swelling, ecchymosis, tenderness and painful range of motion. Median nerve may be injured (13-23% cases) and should be carefully tested. Ipsilateral elbow and shoulder should be examined for associated injuries.

X-rays

Anteroposterior and lateral views of the wrist are usually adequate. X-rays should be evaluated for fracture line, extension, if any, of the fracture into the wrist joint, displacements of the distal radius fragment, status of the distal radio-ulnar joint and the presence of ulnar styloid fracture.

The typical displacements of the distal fragment and comminution are noted (Fig. 9.8).

Treatment

If the fracture is undisplaced or minimally displaced, it is treated in below elbow slab for 6 weeks. Displaced fractures without comminution are treated by manipulation under anaesthesia. Longitudinal traction is applied to disimpact the fracture fragments. This is followed by exaggeration of anterior angulation at the fracture site followed by palmar flexion, ulnar deviation and pronation of distal fragment in one smooth movement. Relative positions of the ulnar (if not fractured) and radial styloid should be compared and below elbow **Colles' cast** is applied (wrist palmar flexed and ulnar deviated). Extreme palmar flexion should be avoided to avoid injury to median nerve.

Check X-rays should be taken immediately following reduction and also weekly for 2 weeks (Fig. 9.12A). If the fracture redisplaces when the swelling comes down, it should be remanipulated or operated. Plaster is worn for 6 weeks and patient is encouraged to move fingers, elbow and shoulder joints during this time.

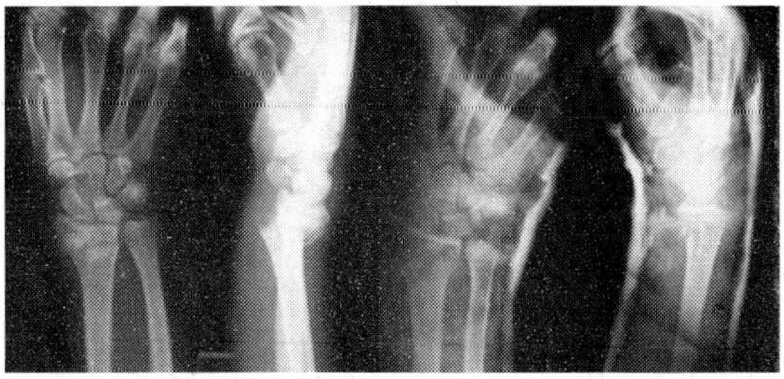

Fig. 9.12A: Pre (left) and post (right) manipulation X rays for Colles' fracture. Note that the normal radiographic relationships have been restored

Intraarticular fractures of the distal end of radius are treated conservatively if they are not widely displaced or extensively comminuted.

Operative treatment is indicated in unstable fractures generally with comminution, or extension inside the wrist joint, where an external fixation

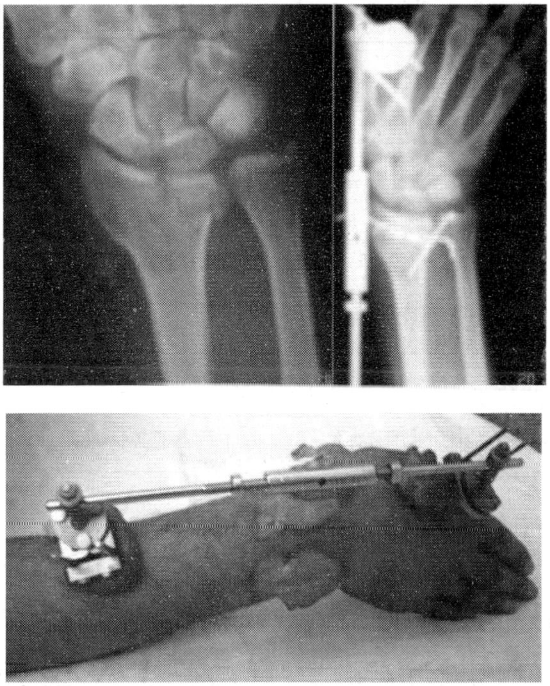

Fig. 9.12B: Comminuted intra articular fracture of distal radius treated by external fixator (Top) X rays; (Bottom) Clinical photograph. Note that Kirschner wires have been used to supplement fixation

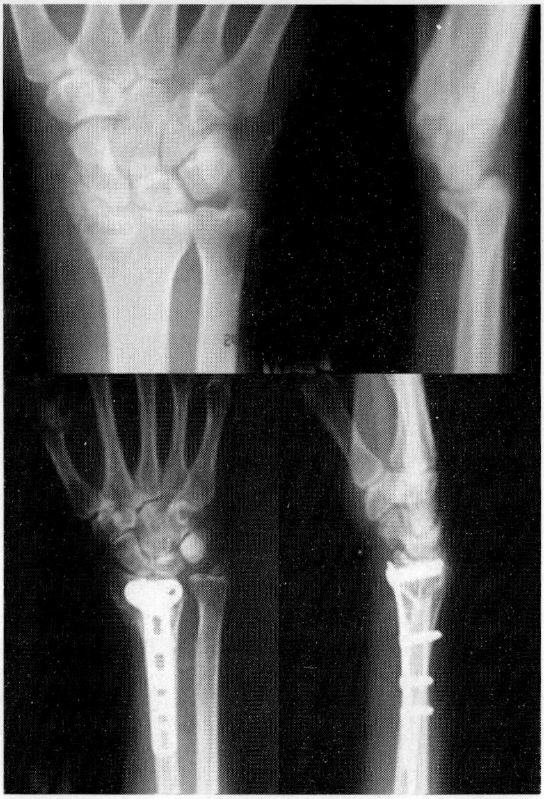

Fig. 9.12C: Comminuted intraarticular volar Barton fracture of distal radius treated by plate and screws (Top) Pre op X-rays; (Bottom) Post Op X-rays

(Fig. 9.12B), fixation with Kirschner wires (supported externally by plaster) or plating with screws can be done (Fig. 9.12C).

Complications

1. Malunion occurs (Fig. 9.13) due to inadequate reduction or immobilization or in extremely comminuted fractures. Manus valgus is commonly seen. Pain may occur on ulnar side of wrist due to ulnar impaction of carpus. In most elderly patients it is accepted. In younger patients it is treated by corrective osteotomy and internal fixation alongwith bone grafting.
2. Stiffness of the fingers, wrist, elbow and hand may occur. Aggressive occupational therapy is

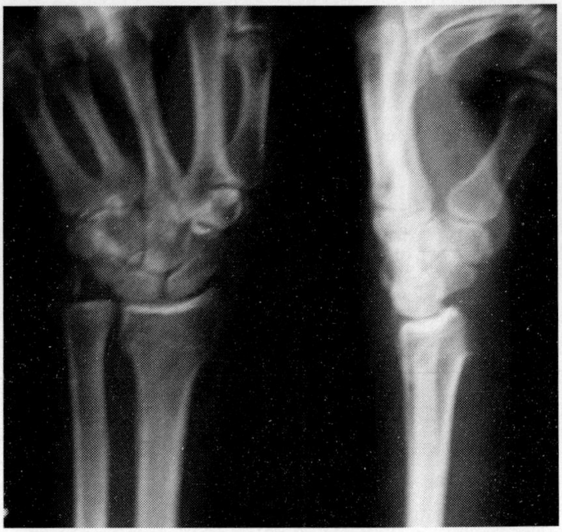

Fig. 9.13: X-rays of malunited Colles' fracture. Note shortening of radius and loss of volar and ulnar tilt of the distal radius articular surface

required to mobilize the joints. All attempts should be made to prevent stiffness.
3. Sudeck's osteodystrophy is reflex sympathetic dystrophy which can be extremely disabling. The hand becomes swollen, discoloured, stiff and hypersensitive. Later on the X-rays show patchy osteoporosis and ground glass appearance of the hand. Early diagnosis, aggressive pain management and physiotherapy and stellate ganglion block (if required) can be useful in reducing morbidity.
4. Subluxation of the radioulnar joint may be persistent if radial shortening is not corrected. The head of the ulna becomes prominent and ulnar side wrist pain and restriction of rotations occurs. Excision of distal end of ulna can be done if the symptoms are disabling.
5. Median nerve injury may occur at the time of fracture or signs of carpal tunnel syndrome may appear after immobilization in extreme palmar flexion or malunion.
6. Tendon rupture, most commonly extensor pollicis longus (EPL) is a rare complication

which may occur a few weeks after the fracture. Treatment is by the transfer of Extensor Indicis to the EPL as the frayed tendon edges are not amenable to repair.

Fractures of the Scaphoid

Scaphoid is the most commonly fractured carpal bone. The scaphoid is completely intrarticular and has no capsular attachments. It receives all its blood supply from distal branches of the radial artery. The fractures of the proximal scaphoid depend on intraosseous blood flow and heal more slowly than distal fractures and have higher rates of non union and avascular necrosis.

Fractures of the scaphoid occur commonly in young men.

Mechanism of Injury and Types

Scaphoid fractures occurs due to fall on the outstretched hand.

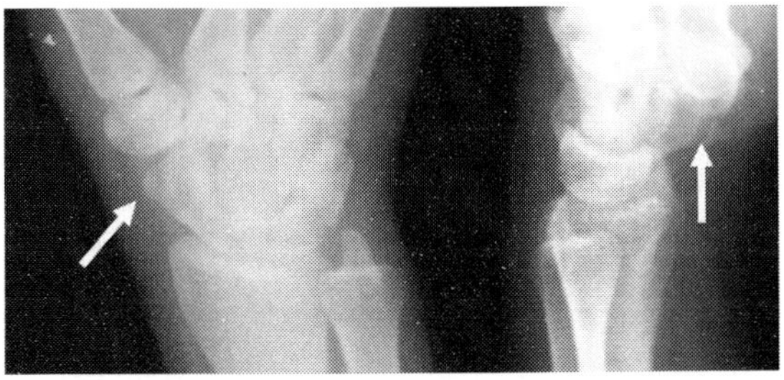

Fig. 9.14A: Fracture of scaphoid tuberosity

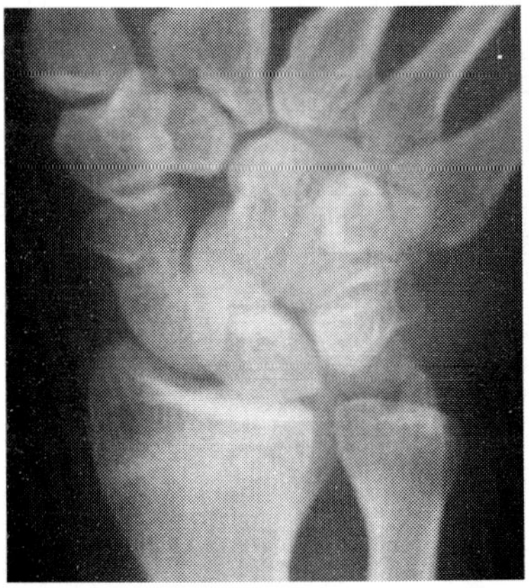

Fig. 9.14B: Fracture of distal third of scaphoid

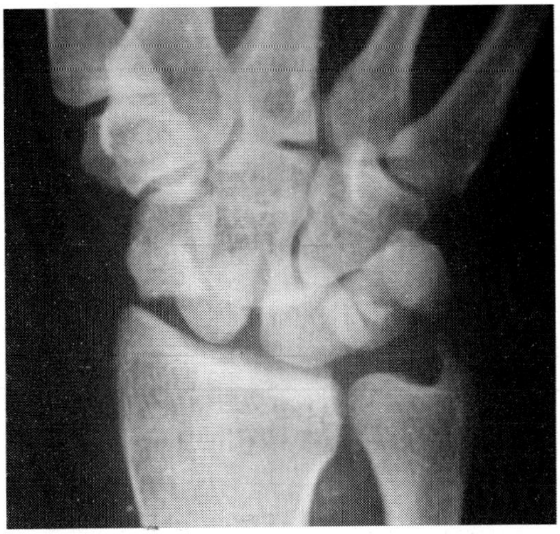

Fig. 9.14C: Fracture of scaphoid waist

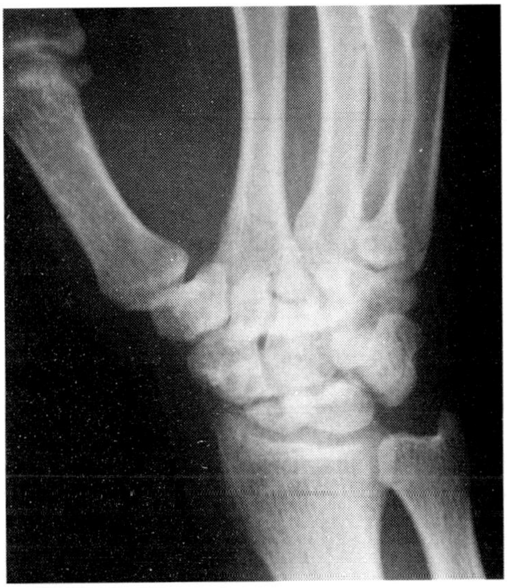

Fig. 9.14D: Fracture of proximal third of scaphoid

Scaphoid fractures are classified according to the location into tuberosity (Fig. 9.14A), distal pole (Fig. 9.14B), waist (Fig. 9.14C) and proximal pole fractures (Fig. 9.14D). Waist fractures are most common (Two thirds).

Clinical Features

Patient presents with history of fall followed by the swelling and tenderness in the anatomical snuff

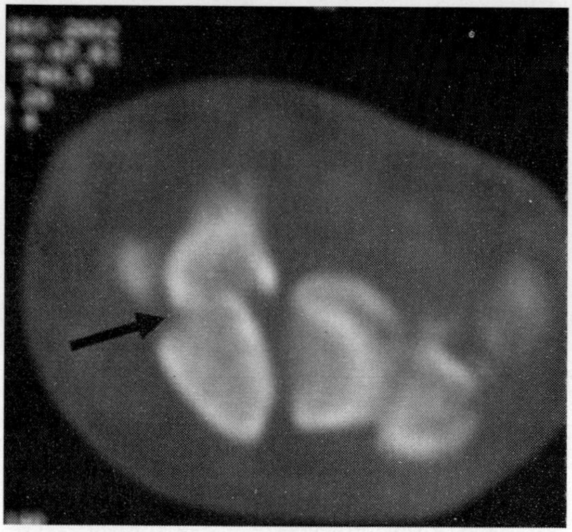

Fig. 9.14E: CT scan showing scaphoid fracture (arrow)

box. Snuff box is the region located at the dorsal aspect of the base of the thumb, between first and second extensor tendon compartments. Resisted pinch between the thumb and index finger is painful and weak.

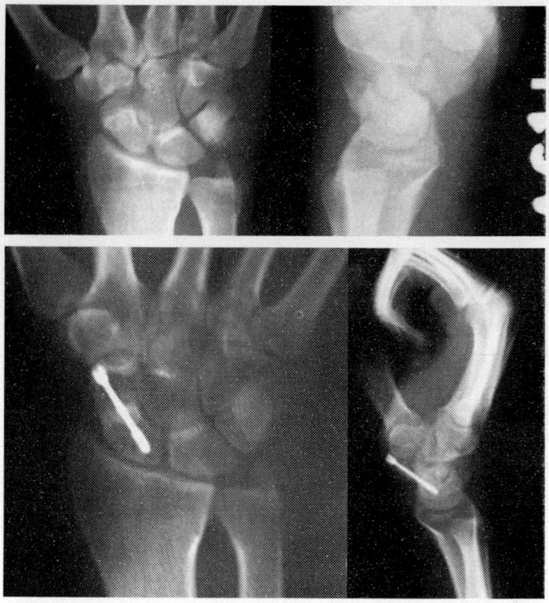

Figs 9.15A and B: Displaced fracture scaphoid treated by headless (Herbert) screw (Top) Pre op (Bottom) Post op X-rays

X-rays

Anteroposterior, lateral and oblique views of the wrist are requisitioned. A scaphoid view (postero-anterior view of the wrist with ulnar deviation) shows scaphoid in profile and is useful when the appearance of scaphoid in other views is equivocal. If X-rays are normal but there is a high index of suspicion, a thumb spica is applied and X-rays repeated out of spica after 2 weeks. The resorption at the ends of the fracture will lead to appearance of fracture line by this time. CT scan (Fig. 9.14E) and MRI are useful imaging modalities for diagnosing scaphoid fractures.

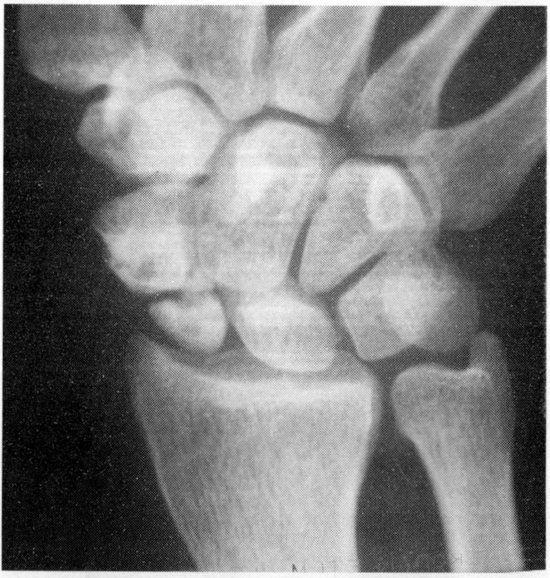

Fig. 9.16: Non union fracture scaphoid. Proximal third fractures are most prone to undergo non union. Note the sclerotic fracture ends and gap at fracture site.

Treatment

Undisplaced fractures are treated in a short arm thumb spica cast for 6 to 12 weeks. Proximal pole fractures heal more slowly (12-24 weeks). Displaced fractures (displaced more than 1 mm) are treated operatively. Anatomic reduction of scaphoid and fixation with K wires or Herbert (head less) screw is performed (Fig. 9.15).

Complications

1. Non union (Fig. 9.16): Occurs in 5 to 10% but is nearly 90% in displaced proximal pole fractures. Failure to heal in 6 months establishes non union. Treatment is by cancellous bone grafting with or without internal fixation.
2. *Malunion:* With apex dorsal deformity; it may need osteotomy and bone grafting in a young patient.
3. Avascular necrosis occurs due to precarious blood supply of scaphoid and is seen in 90% to 100% cases of scaphoid fracture in the proximal fifth.
4. *Post traumatic arthritis:* Occurs due to malunion, non union or avascular necrosis of the scaphoid.
5. Instability of the carpus may occur after a scaphoid fracture.

Fractures of the Other Carpal Bones

Scaphoid is followed in incidence by the lunate and triquetral. Fractures of the other carpal bones are rare.

Dislocation of the Lunate

Lunate is the most commonly dislocated bone in the carpus. It is believed to follow perilunate dislocation (see below) where the lunate remains in place and the rest of the carpus dislocates. When the carpus snaps back, it may lever luante out of its articulation with radius.

Mechanisms of Injury and Types

A fall on the outstretched hand with forced dorsiflexion is the causative injury. The dislocation is usually anterior.

Clinically, the patient presents with painful and swollen wrist and inability to move the wrist. If dislocated lunate compresses the median nerve anteriorly, there may be signs of median nerve dysfunction.

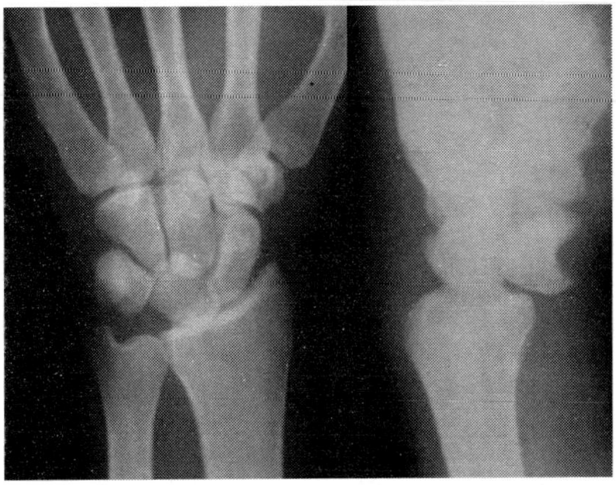

Fig. 9.17: Volar dislocation of lunate

X-rays Anteroposterior and lateral views of the wrist are taken. The anteroposterior view shows decreased height of the carpus. Lateral view is diagnostic and shows a lunate which is tilted forward and is no more articulating with the distal radius. It lies in front of the wrist and is rotated 90° or more on the horizontal axis so that its concave distal articular surface faces volarwards (Fig. 9.17).

Treatment of lunate dislocation is reduction under anaesthesia. Strong traction is applied to the dorsiflexed hand and while maintaining traction, wrist is palmarflexed while lunate is pushed backwards by the other hand. Reduction occurs when lunate pops back in position. A below elbow plaster cast is applied for 4 weeks.

Open reduction is performed if closed reduction fails. Anterior approach is commonly used, carpal tunnel is decompressed and the reduction is maintained by Kirschner wires.

Complications include median nerve injury, irreducible dislocation and high incidence of stiffness and degenerative joint disease of the wrist. Avascular necrosis of the lunate may occur as all its soft tissue attachments are disrupted.

Perilunate Dislocation

In perilunate dislocations, lunate remains in place while the rest of the carpus dislocates dorsally

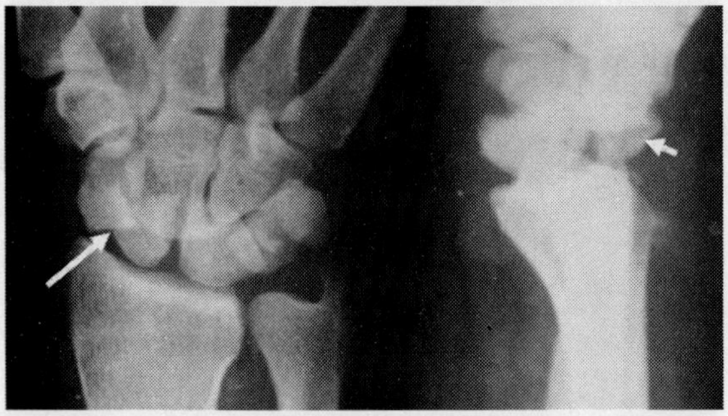

Fig. 9.18: Perilunate dislocation. Note that the lunate retains its normal articulation with radius while capitate and the rest of the carpus have dislocated dorsally (short arrow). Also note that the scaphoid has fractured along the waist (long arrow)

(Fig. 9.18). It is also caused by the fall on the outstretched hand. Clinically, the patient presents with pain and swelling over dorsal aspect of the wrist. Lateral radiograph of the wrist shows normal relationship of lunate with radius while the rest of the carpus is displaced dorsal to the wrist. Treatment is reduction under anaesthesia using traction in dorsiflexion and then trying to push proximal capitate along the dorsal lip of lunate, in the distal articular concavity of the lunate. This maneuver can sometimes convert a perilunate dislocation into lunate dislocation. Failure of closed reduction is indication for open reduction of the dislocation.

INJURIES OF THE HAND

Hand injuries are common and lead to significant disability. It is the judgment of the doctor who first manages the patient that decides the final outcome. It is, therefore, extremely important to examine all hand injuries carefully and plan treatment meticulously.

The following principles must be observed while managing hand injuries:

1. Circulation must be carefully assessed in all hand injuries.
2. Neurologic function should be assessed by testing motor and sensory components of median, ulnar and radial nerves.
3. Integrity of the tendons should be assessed by asking the patient to move his fingers.
4. On flexion, digits 2 to 5 point towards the tubercle of scaphoid. A rotational deformity exists if they do not.
5. Fingers joints should be immobilized for the minimal period required to avoid stiffness.
6. In general, hand should be splinted in the position of safe immobilization wherein the metacarpo-phalangeal joints are flexed 70° to 90°, the finger joints are extended and the thumb is abducted. In this position, the ligaments of the respective joints are stretched to their longest and stiffness is least likely.
7. Fracture lines in hand bones may be visible on plain X-rays for even one year following injury and this alone should not be taken as proof of non union. It is standard care to discard immobilization and mobilize hand joints after 3 weeks.

Common Fractures in the Hand

Metacarpal Fractures

Metacarpal fractures can occur at the base, in the shaft or through the neck (Fig. 9.19). These are caused by falls or blow on the hand. Metacarpal fractures may result in shortening thus leading to loss of prominence of the knuckle. Oblique fractures tend to shorten while the spiral fractures tend to rotate. Undisplaced fractures of the metacarpals are treated in a dorsal slab for 3 weeks.

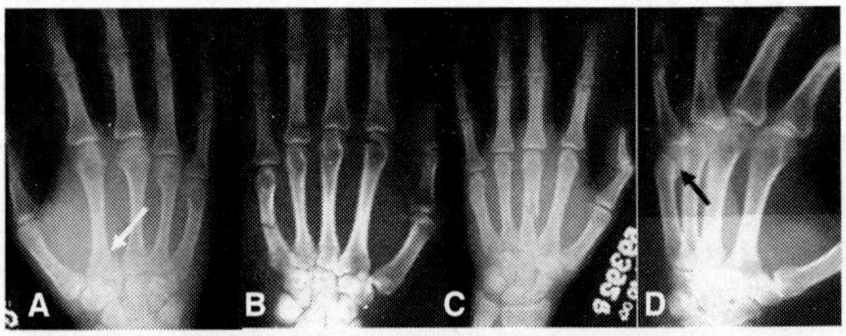

Fig. 9.19: Metacarpal fractures (A) Base of second metacarpal (white arrow) (B) Shaft of 5th metacarpal (C) Shaft of third metacarpal (D) Neck of 5th metacarpal (black arrow)

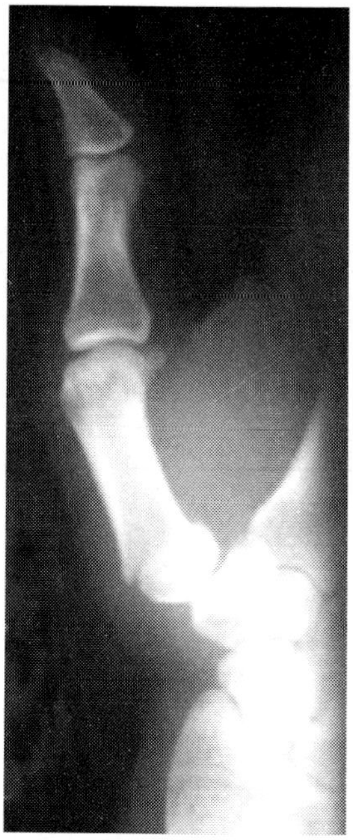

Fig. 9.20: Extra articular fracture base of thumb metacarpal

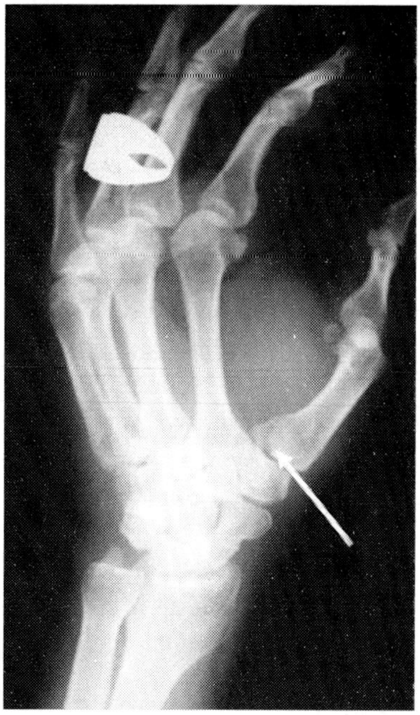

Fig. 9.21: Bennett's fracture dislocation. Note the typical triangular medial fragment (arrow)

For the displaced fractures, reduction followed by the use of K wire, circumferential wire, screws or screws with small plate to fix the fracture is undertaken. The fourth and fifth metacarpals are more mobile than second and third and thus can compensate for more residual deformity (20-30° as compared to 10° for 2nd and 3rd). Rotational malunion leads to overlap of digits in flexion.

Fractures of the Thumb Metacarpal

Fractures of the thumb metacarpal occur commonly near the base and can be extra articular (Fig. 9.20) or intra-articular. Fractures are usually sustained during boxing or punching. The extra articular fracture is usually impacted and stable. The intra-articular fracture can be an oblique fracture entering the carpometacarpal joint with proximal displacement of the distal fragment (Bennett's fracture—subluxation) or a comminuted T or Y intra-articular fracture of the base of first metacarpal (Rolando's fracture) (Fig. 9.21 and 9.22).

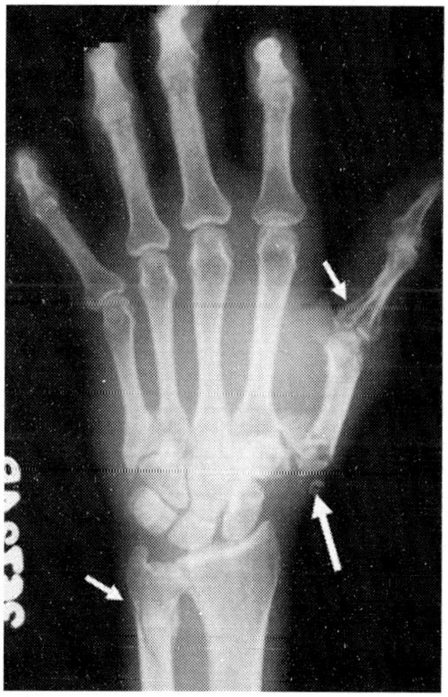

Fig. 9.22: Intraarticular comminuted fracture of the base of first metacarpal (long arrow). Also note the comminuted fractures of base of proximal phalanx of thumb and ulna (short arrows)

Bennett's fracture subluxation is an unstable fracture. Patient presents with shortening of the thumb and swelling in the region of the carpometacarpal joint. X-rays reveal a small volar ulnar triangular fragment that retains its articulation with medial trapezium while the combined pull of abductors and adductors of the thumb pulls the proximal fragment proximally and into adduction.

Although these fractures can be almost always reduced by closed means, they are unstable and it is difficult to maintain reduction. The fracture is reduced under anaesthesia by traction on thumb metacarpal followed by abduction and extension of the thumb. This position can then be maintained by well moulded plater cast or by Kirschner wire or a screw. Check X-rays should be taken in case plaster alone is being relied upon to maintain the reduction. Immobilization is continued for 4 weeks.

Complications

1. Malunion: due to inability to achieve or maintain reduction.
2. Osteoarthritis occurs due to damage to the joint and/or imperfect reduction of the articular surface. (That is the reason why perfect reduction should be aimed in the intra-articular fractures).

Fracture of the Neck of the Fifth Metacarpal (Boxer's Fracture)

Boxer's fracture is any impacted fracture of the neck of the fifth metacarpal sustained by a direct blow with a closed fist. There is local pain and swelling following injury and X-rays show a transverse fracture of the neck of fifth metacarpal with dorsal angulation and head of metacarpal tilted in the palm (Fig. 9.23).

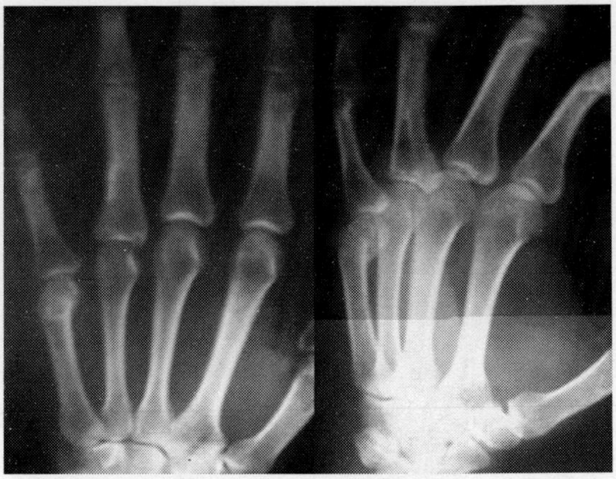

Fig. 9.23: Fracture neck of fifth metacarpal. Note the dorsal angulation and tilt of metacarpal head in palm

Treatment

Due to the mobility of the fifth metacarpal, upto 40° angulation can be accepted (Only 20° is acceptable in the index and middle metacarpal neck fractures). Therefore, treatment consists of correcting any rotational deformity and immobilization in a splint or ball bandage for 3 weeks. The fractures are often unstable and tend to redisplace in which case percutaneous K wires can be used to fix these fractures.

Complications

Malunion leads to a prominent metacarpal head in the palm and pseudo clawing (Z appearance) as metacarpophalangeal joint hyperextends to compensate for the deformity.

Fractures of the Phalanges

Fractures of the phalanges usually occur due to direct injuries and are often compound. Phalangeal fractures may occur at the base (intra-or extra articular), shaft, neck or in the condyles (Fig. 9.24). Phalangeal fractures always unite whether immobilized or not. Displaced intra articular and unstable diaphyseal fractures should be fixed using cerclage wires, K wires or screws (Fig. 9.25). Undisplaced or stable fracture are treated by buddy splinting wherein the injured finger is strapped to its neighbours (buddy)—uninjured finger and movements are encouraged to avoid stiffness. Splintage is discontinued at 3 weeks.

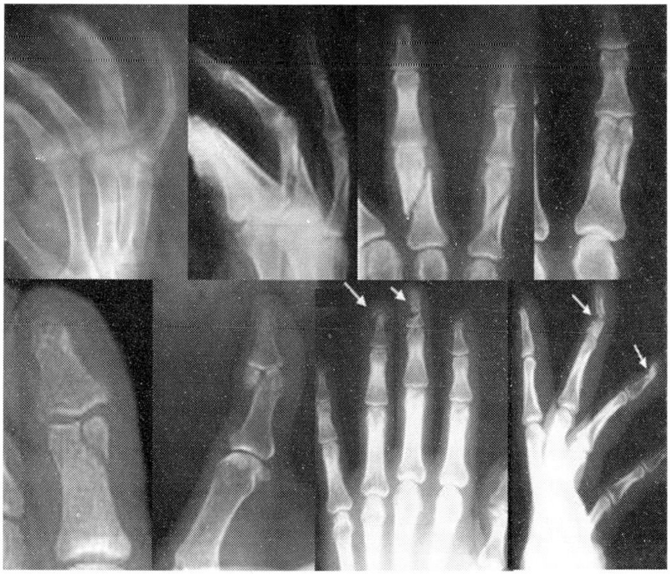

Fig. 9.24: Phalangeal fracture: different sites and fracture configurations

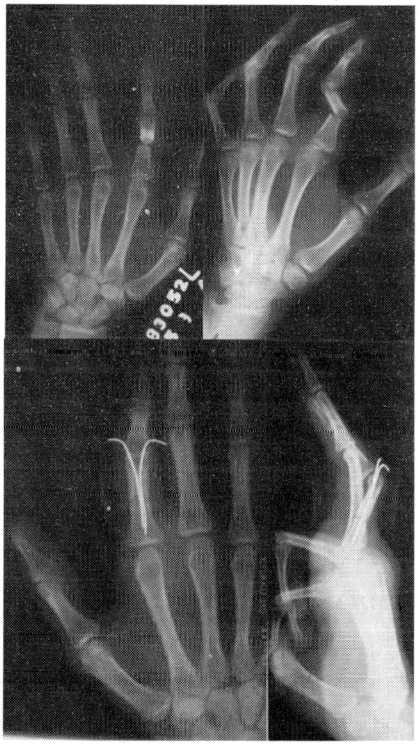

Fig. 9.25: Unstable phalangeal fracture (Top) treated with internal fixation (Bottom)

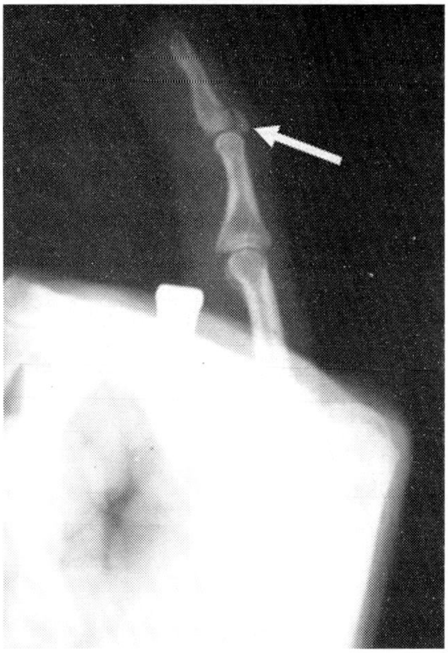

Fig. 9.26: Mallet finger. Note the avulsion of bony attachment (arrow) of the extensor tendon at the base of distal phalanx

Mallet Finger (Also called Baseball Fracture)

Mallet finger occurs when sudden passive flexion of the distal interphalangeal joint leads to avulsion of the extensor tendon insertion from the base of the distal phalanx of the finger (Fig. 9.26). Sometimes the extensor tendon may rupture at its insertion. The distal phalanx cannot extend, hence its slightly flexed attitude is termed mallet finger. Treatment of bony avulsion is by open reduction and fixation by wire or wire suture. Tendon avulsion is treated by splintage in a Mallet finger splint for 6 weeks maintaining distal interphalangeal joint in hyperextension.

Dislocations of the Hand Joints

Metacarpophalangeal Joint Dislocations

Occur due to hyper extension injury. Proximal phalanx is prominent over dorsal aspect of the finger. Lateral X-ray of the affected finger clinches

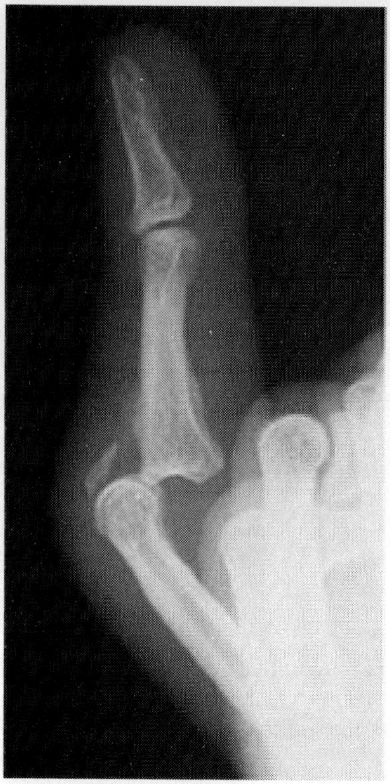

Fig. 9.27: Metacarpophlangeal joint dislocation of thumb

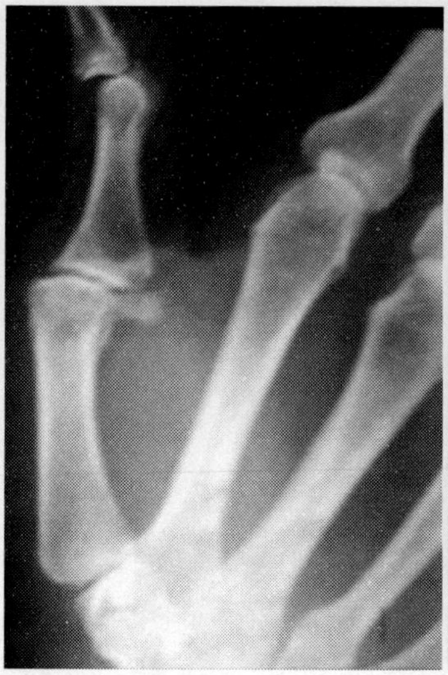

Fig. 9.28: Dislocation of interphalangeal joint of the thumb

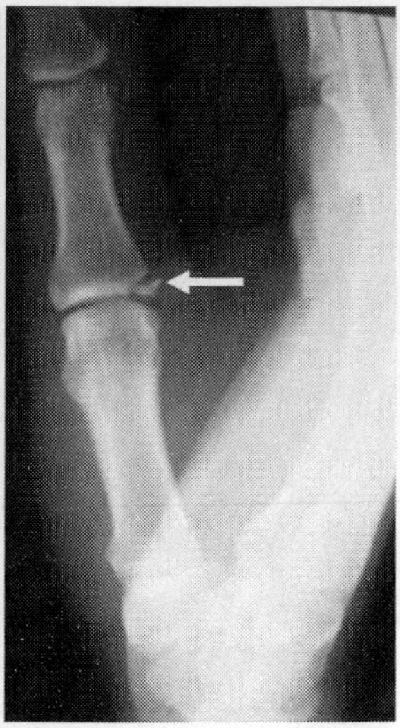

Fig. 9.29: Gamekeeper's thumb. Note the bony flake avulsed (arrow) by the ulnar collateral ligament attachment

the diagnosis (Fig. 9.27). Treatment is by closed reduction which is achieved by hyperextending the MP joint and then gradually flexing it while metacarpal is pushed back by the other hand. Following reduction immobilization is continued in 50° flexion at the metacarpophalangeal joint for 3 weeks. Sometimes the metacarpal head "button holes" through a rent in the front of capsule and these "complex" dislocations cannot be reduced by closed means. Open reduction is undertaken and volar capsule is divided to bring the metacarpal head back and reduce the joint.

Interphalangeal Joint Dislocations

Interphalangeal joint dislocations (Fig. 9.28) are more common in proximal interphalangeal joints. These commonly occur due to hyper extension injury and are easily reduced by pulling. Following reduction, buddy splinting is continued for 2-3 weeks.

Game Keeper's Thumb (Skier's thumb)

Forceful hyper abduction (radial deviation) of the thumb leads to tearing of ulnar collateral ligament of the first metacarpophalangeal joint. Tear may be partial or complete. A small bony flake may be avulsed at times (Fig. 9.29). Patient presents with pain, tenderness and swelling over ulnar aspect of thumb MP joint. There is inability to perform pinching activities. If not treated appropriately, the condition leads to chronic instability.

Treatment

Partial tears are treated by 3 weeks of immobilization in a cast or splint followed by physiotherapy. Complete tears are surgically repaired followed by immobilization in a thumb spica for 4 weeks.

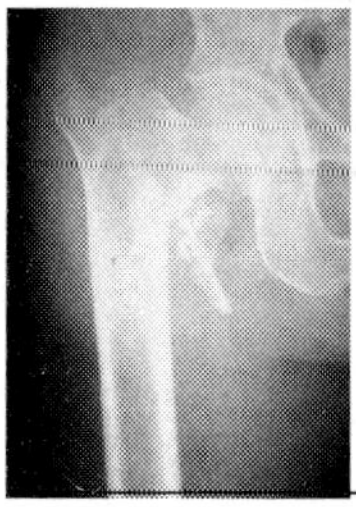

10 Fractures of the Pelvis and Hip

Pelvis fractures, Hip dislocation, Femoral neck fractures, Intertrochanteric fractures, Slipped capital femoral epiphysis

Fractures of the pelvis can occur following the injuries of varying severity. In young patients, these fracture occurs with severe high-energy injuries while in old patients with osteoporosis, these injuries can occur following a trivial, low-energy fall.

The most important aspects of the pelvis fractures especially high energy ones are:

1. Treat there injuries with respect.
   a. They have high morbidity and mortality.
   b. They have high incidence of associated injuries to:
      - rest of skeleton
      - urogenital system
      - chest
      - viscera/abdomen
2. Hemorrhage (especially in the retroperitoneum) is the single most important cause of death in these patients.
3. Pelvis X-rays **must** be routinely taken in **all** patients with polytrauma or severe injuries to the lower extremity. These fractures have a reputation for being missed. Have a high index of suspicion.
4. The urethra in males is longer and thus more prone to injury following pelvis fractures than in females. The most common part of urethra injured is membranous part and the most common fracture pattern associated with urethral injury is **straddle** fracture (Bilateral superior and inferior pubic rami fractures).
5. All pelvis fracture patients **must** be hospitalized.

Mechanism of Injury and Types

Mechanism of injury for low energy injury can be sudden muscular contraction in young athletes (leading to avulsion fracture) or domestic falls (leading to isolated pubic ramus or straddle type fracture). High energy injuries can disrupt the pelvis by the anteroposterior compression, lateral compression or the vertical shear injuries or a combination.

The pelvis factures can be classified as stable or unstable. **Stable** fractures are defined as those which can withstand normal physiological forces without abnormal deformation i.e. these fractures do not seriously disrupt the integrity of the pelvic ring. These include isolated (avulsion) fractures of anterior superior iliac spine (due to pull of sartorius), anterior inferior iliac spine (pull of rectus femoris), or ischial tuberosity (pull of hamstrings). Also, fractures with a **single** break in the pelvic ring (such as fracture of the superior or inferior pubic ramus or of both the rami on the same side; fracture of the wing of ilium from direct violence) are inherently stable (Fig. 10.1).

Unstable fractures are said to occur when the integrity of the pelvic ring is seriously disrupted and the pelvis cannot withstand normal physiological forces without abnormal deformation. Generally speaking, fractures or dislocations with disruption of the pelvic ring at two points are unstable. For example, disruption of symphysis pubis with fracture of sacrum (Fig. 10.2) or fracture of superior and inferior pubic ramus with

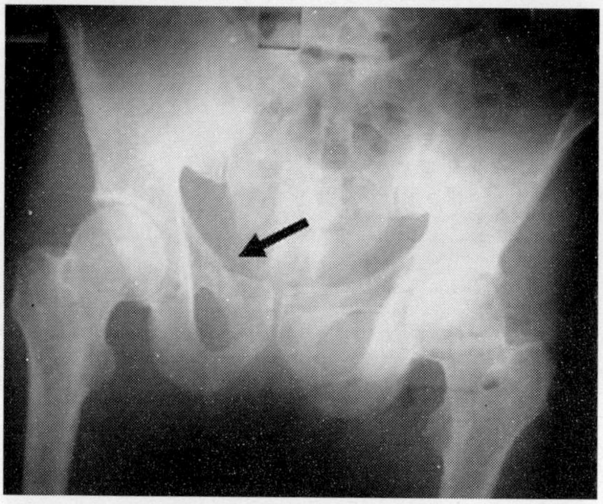

Fig. 10.1: Stable pelvis fracture. Single break in pelvic ring—Right superior pubic ramus fracture (arrow)

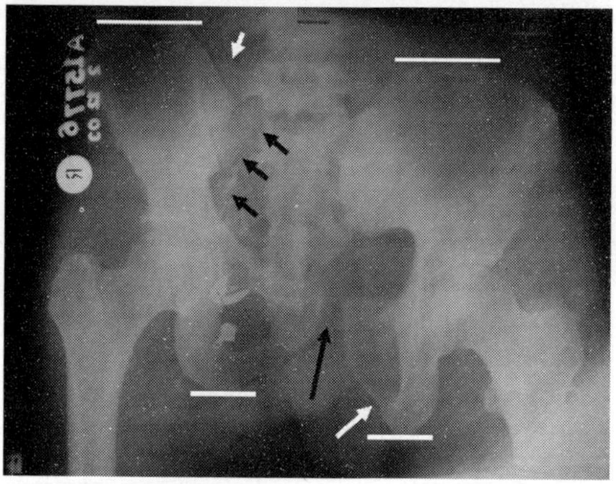

Fig. 10.2: Unstable pelvis fracture. Pelvic ring broken at more than one places (arrows)—Disruption of pubic symphysis, fracture of inferior pubic ramus, fracture of sacrum and fracture of the right L_5 transverse process. Note that the right half of pelvis is riding up (compare levels of ischial tuberosities and iliac crests)

dislocation of sacro-iliac joints or any other combination are the examples of the unstable pelvic fractures.

Clinical Features

Clinical evaluation of the patient with pelvis fracture must begin with assessment of the patient including **A**irway, **B**reathing, **C**irculation, and **D**isability.

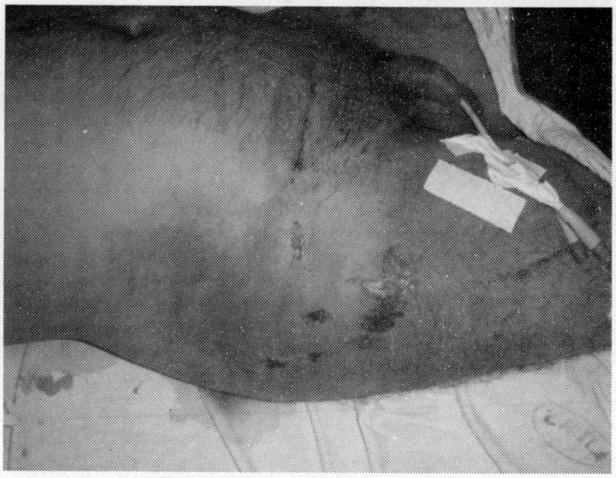

Fig. 10.3: Massive contusions with pelvis fracture suggest significant bleeding. These patients have associated severe soft tissue injuries

Resuscitation must be started immediately and life threatening injuries addressed. Injuries to head, chest, abdomen, spine and extremities should be evaluated. Clinical signs of pelvis fracture include asymmetry of the legs, pain in the pelvis, pain on hip movements and, with anterior pelvis fractures, swelling and local tenderness at the symphysis. Pelvis compression test is positive (elicits pain). Massive flank or buttock contusions (Fig. 10.3) and swelling with hemorrhage are indicative of significant bleeding. Palpation of symphysis may reveal a defect while palpation of the posterior aspect of pelvic may reveal a hematoma or a defect due to sacral fracture or sacro-iliac dislocation. Perineum must be carefully inspected for wound(s) and a per rectal in all and per vaginal examination in females must be performed in all patients. Hemodynamic status must be monitored and neurologic injury must be assessed. High index of suspicion must be maintained for genitourinary and gastrointestinal injuries. Retention of urine, blood at the meatus, perineal hematoma and high riding or "floating" prostate at per rectal examination all suggest urethral injuries which are seen in nearly 10% cases. Rupture of the bladder can occur in nearly 20% cases. A bowel loop trapped at the fracture site may present with gastro intestinal obstruction.

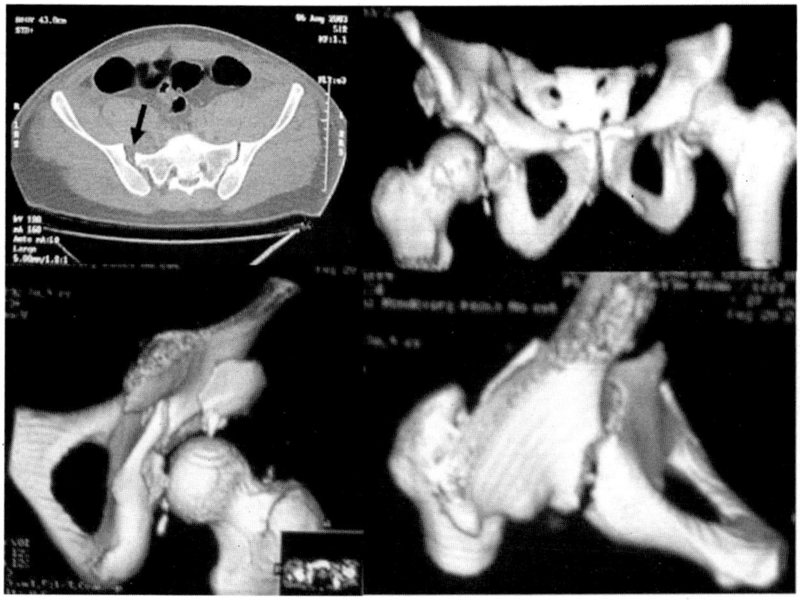

Fig. 10.4: CT scan. (Top left) is very useful for evaluating sacrum fractures and sacro-iliac joint injuries (arrow). 3D reconstruction scans (Top right, Bottom) show the fracture fragments and displacements

X-rays: A plain anteroposterior X-ray of the pelvis is able to give most of the required information about a pelvis fracture. However, inlet and outlet views of the pelvis can be taken for additional information. A CT scan can effectively demonstrate the injury to the posterior ring (sacrum fracture, SI joint disruption) (Fig. 10.4). A FAST (Focussed Assessment of Sonography for Trauma) ultrasound assessment is now known to the more efficient than DPL (Diagnostic Peritoneal Lavage) for detecting intra-abdominal injuries. A retrograde urethrogram should be done in cases where a urethral injury is suspected/present.

Treatment

Stable pelvis fractures are treated with protected weight bearing and symptomatic treatment.

Treatment of the unstable pelvis fractures is difficult and determined by the associated injuries and the hemodynamic status of the patient. Hemodynamic stabilization often requires reducing the volume of the pelvis and producing tamponade by tying a sheet or brace around pelvis or applying an external fixator. An external fixator can be definitive treatment for diastasis of pubic symphysis seen in open book (anteroposterior compression) injuries (Fig. 10.5). Internal fixation of the unstable pelvic ring (with plates and screws) is sometimes undertaken for displaced iliac wing fractures, diastasis of symphysis pubis, and sacro-iliac dislocations. Sometimes long (iliosacral) screws are used to fix the sacroiliac joint after reducing the dislocation.

Complications

1. Exsanguinating hemorrhage is managed by fluid resuscitation, blood replacement, achieving temponade by sheet, brace or external fixator and angiography followed by embolization/direct repair in case of vascular injuries.
2. Urogenital injuries are common and are treated on their merits. Urethral injuries are treated by suprapubic cystostomy followed by urethral repair at a subsequent time.
3. Injuries to viscera (solid as well as hollow viscus) and rupture of the diaphragm can occur.
4. Infection may occur in 0% to 25% especially in open injuries and following operative repair of posterior injuries.
5. Nerve injuries. Displacement of the SI joint or fracture of the sacrum may lead to injury to the lumbosacral plexus.

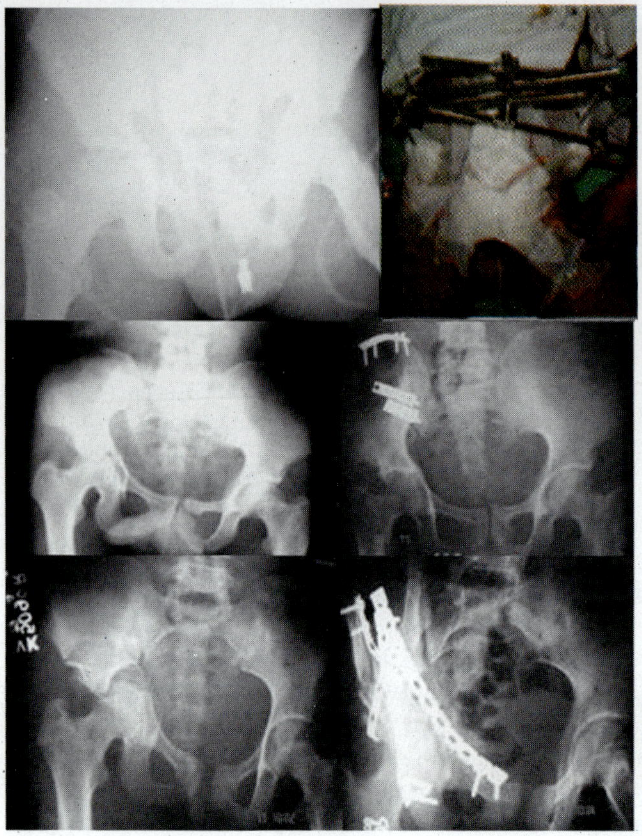

Fig. 10.5: Treatment of unstable pelvis fracture (Top left) can be by external fixator (Top right) or internal fixation. (Middle and Bottom rows) Fracture involving acetabulum treated by multiple plates and screws

6. Thromboembolism can occur following deep vein thrombosis (DVT).
7. Malunion and non union can lead to pain, gait abnormalities, sitting difficulties, low back pain, pelvic outlet obstruction and nerve root irritation.
8. Impotence can occur following pelvis fractures.

Dislocations and Fracture-Dislocations of the Hip

Hip dislocations are orthopedic emergencies and are the only skeletal injuries which take precedence over management of head injuries. The following facts should be remembered about the hip dislocations:

a. Hip dislocations are painful and may lead to persistent shock if not treated urgently.
b. Always get an AP X-ray of pelvis in major lower extremity fractures to rule out hip dislocation.

   Remember: In dashboard injuries, femur shaft fractures and knee injuries share the same mechanism of injury as the posterior hip dislocation.
c. In femoral shaft fractures proximal fragment is abducted. An adducted proximal fragment should raise the suspicion of coexistent hip dislocation.
d. Sciatic nerve injury is present in 8% to 19% cases of posterior dislocation of hip due to its close proximity to hip. Always look for sciatic nerve function in hip dislocation.
e. The longer the hip remains dislocated, higher the risk of avascular necrosis of the femoral head.
f. CT scan is often required for irreducible hips, hips which are not concentrically reduced or unstable hips. While inability to achieve

concentric reduction is due to interposition of a fragment, unstable hips are due to associated large posterior lip fragments.

g. The hip joint is anatomically strong and considerable violence is needed to dislocate the hip.

Mechanism of Injury and Types

Posterior dislocations are the commonest with the anterior dislocations constituting 10% to 15% of the cases. These injuries are commonly caused by high velocity trauma, mostly motor vehicle accidents, fall from height or industrial accidents. In head-on-collision car accidents the front seat traveller strikes his knee to the dashboard and force transmission along the thigh (flexed at hip as in sitting position) dislocates the hip posteriorly. Such "dashboard injuries" may also cause fracture of patella, fracture of femur shaft or cruciate ligament injuries at the knee. Anterior dislocation occurs when the dislocating force is applied to the posterior pelvis with the ipsilateral foot or knee acting as the counter force. Hip dislocation may be classified according to the direction of displacement of the femoral head such as anterior, posterior or central (medial). Hip dislocation may be simple or fracture dislocation (when associated with fracture of the acetabulum or the femoral head).

Clinical Features

Examination to rule out associated severe injuries to spine, chest, head, abdomen etc. should be performed in all cases. The position of the leg is often an indicator of hip dislocation:

Posterior dislocation: The leg is held in flexion, adduction and internal rotation (Fig. 10.6).

Anterior dislocation: The leg is held in external rotation, abduction and some flexion (Fig. 10.7).

It is often possible to feel a fullness in the soft tissues in the direction of displacement of head;

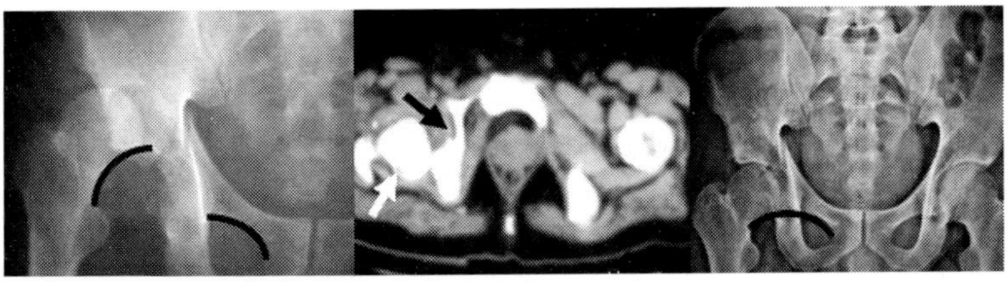

Fig. 10.6: Posterior dislocation of right hip. (Left) Note that the femur is up ridden, there is loss of congruence between the femoral head and acetabulum. Shenton's line is broken. (Middle) Axial CT cuts show that femoral head (white arrow) is dislocated posteriorly while the acetabulum (black arrow) is empty. CT is very useful for demonstrating associated fractures of femoral head and acetabulum and for intra-articular bony fragments. (Right) AP X-ray after reduction of dislocation. Note that the Shenton's line is restored

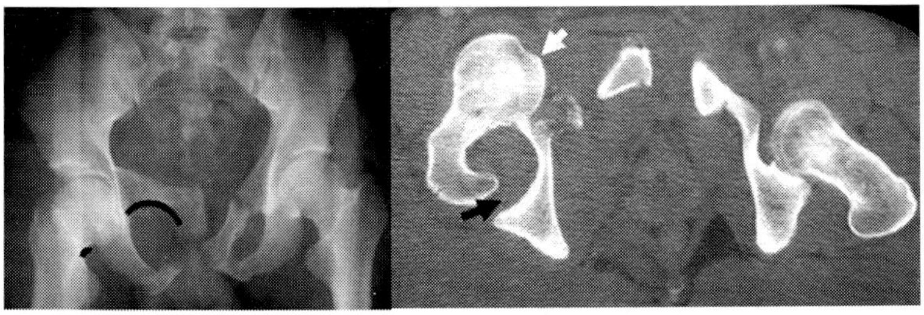

Fig. 10.7: Anterior dislocation right hip. (Left) Note that the Shenton's line is broken. (Right) CT scan-axial cut showing femoral head (white arrow) dislocated anteriorly and empty acetabulum (black arrow)

this bony fullness rotates when rotation of distal limb is attempted, confirming it to be femoral head (Remember: This maneuver is very painful!).

Neurovascular examination must be done in all cases. Peroneal distribution of the sciatic nerve is involved more often. A posterior dislocation of hip makes anterior palpation of the femoral pulsations difficult (Narath sign).

X-rays: An anteroposterior (AP) radiograph of the pelvis, as well as a cross-table lateral of the affected hip is essential.

Plain X-rays are evaluated for femoral head size on the two sides, symmetry, joint spaces and Shenton's line (Fig. 10.6). Appearance of the lesser trochanter indicates pathologic internal or external rotation of the limb. Femoral head depression and fractures as well as acetabular fractures may be seen.

CT scan is indicated for hips which are irreducible or not concentrically reduced to rule out intraarticular fragments.

MRI may prove helpful to evaluate vascularity of the femoral head.

Treatment

Reduction should be expedient to reduce the risk of avascular necrosis which worsens significantly if the reduction is delayed for more than 12 hours.

An immediate closed reduction under general anaesthesia should be attempted in all cases. The commonly used techniques for posterior dislocation of the hip are as follows:

1. Allis Method

The patient is supine, preferably on the floor or low couch. The traction is applied in line with the deformity while the assistant applies counter traction by stabilizing the pelvis. While increasing the traction force, the surgeon slowly increases the degree of flexion to approximately 70°. Gentle internal rotation and adduction is done. With maximal traction, the leg is gently rotated in internal and external rotation to help the femoral head clear the lip of the acetabulum. The reduction is dramatic with an audible "clunk" and is stabilized by external rotation, extension and abduction.

2. Stimson Gravity Method

The patient is placed prone with the affected hip flexed 90° off the side of the stretcher. The ipsilateral knee is bent 90° and force is applied to the back of the proximal calf. Gentle rotation of the limb may assist in reduction.

Caution: The prone technique is contraindicated in patients with multiple trauma.

3. Bigelow Method

The patient is supine and the surgeon applies longitudinal traction to the limb. The adducted and internally rotated thigh is then flexed at least 90°. The femoral head is levered into the acetabulum by abduction, external rotation and extension of the hip.

Caution: This method has been associated with iatrogenic femoral neck fractures!

Technique for Reduction of Anterior Dislocation of Hip

The anterior dislocations are harder to reduce than posterior. With the leg in external rotation, abduction and flexion, in line traction is applied. The leg is rocked in internal and external rotation to allow femoral head to negotiate the anterior acetabular rim. Direct pressure over the femoral head in inguinal region is often helpful in forcing the head back into the joint.

Treatment Following Reduction

Following reduction the stability of the hip is checked through the range of motion.

A post reduction CT scan should be done in all cases. A CT scan shows symmetry of reduction, incarcerated bony fragments, if any, and predicts stability (posterior acetabular fragments including >50% posterior wall suggest instability).

If hip is stable it is treated with short period of bed rest followed by protected weight bearing for 4 to 6 weeks.

If hip is unstable, it is treated by skeletal traction for 6 to 8 weeks followed by progressive protected weight bearing.

Open reduction is indicated for:

- Irreducible dislocation
- Non concentric reduction
- Ipsilateral femoral neck fracture
- Associated fracture of acetabulum or femoral head that requires surgery.

Prognosis

A functional outcome with good or excellent result is seen in 70% to 80% cases. Dislocations with associated acetabular, femoral head or femoral neck fractures have poor prognosis.

Complications

1. Sciatic nerve injury (8-19% cases) due to stretching of nerve by the dislocated head. Prognosis is unpredictable though 40-50% incidence of full recovery is reported.
2. Avascular necrosis of the femoral head is seen in 5%-40% cases with higher risk with increased duration of dislocation before reduction (>6 to 24 hours).
3. Post traumatic arthritis: especially when associated with femoral head fractures, acetabular fractures or avascular necrosis.
4. Heterotopic ossification (Myositis ossificans) has been reported in 2% cases.
5. Thromboembolism may occur.

Fractures of the Upper End of Femur

Fractures at the upper end of femur are essentially injuries of the elderly and the bones are often osteoporotic. These injuries are more common in females. Also, as these fractures occur in the elderly, medical problems are often associated.

Femoral Neck Fractures

Femoral neck fractues are intra capsular fractures that occur in the proximal femur. Femoral neck extends from the distal extent of the femoral head to the proximal most extent of the inter trochanteric region. An intra capsular fracture can cut off the blood supply to the femoral head completely leading to avascular necrosis, non union or both.

Mechanism of Injury and Types

Older people sustain femoral neck fractures as a result of trivial fall. The young individuals sustain these fractures as a result of high-energy injuries and may have associated femoral shaft fractures or hip dislocations as well as injuries to head, chest or abdomen. The femoral neck fracture are divided according to the location of fracture line into subcapital, transcervical and basicervical (Fig. 10.8). Pauwel classified femoral neck fractures according to the angle that the fracture line makes with the horizontal plane. Type I forms angle upto 30°, Type II forms 30-50° (Fig. 10.9) and Type III forms angle more than 50°.

With increasing angles, there are increasing shearing forces across the fracture site.

The femoral neck fractures can also be classified as undisplaced (impacted) or displaced.

Clinical Features

Patients with acute hip fractures are typically unable to ambulate with shortening and external rotation of the lower extremity. The range of movements is painful and groin is tender on palpation. In undisplaced fractures the obvious deformities are absent but groin tenderness and pain on range of motion are present.

X-rays

An anteroposterior view with hip in internal rotation and a cross-table lateral view should be obtained. AP X-rays reveal break in the femoral neck, upriding of greater trochanter and break in Shenton's line. In case of high suspicion of undisplaced femoral neck fracture when X-rays are normal, an MRI may detect femoral neck fracture. Similarly Tc^{99m} bone scan, performed 48 hours after injury may rule out or diagnose occult fracture.

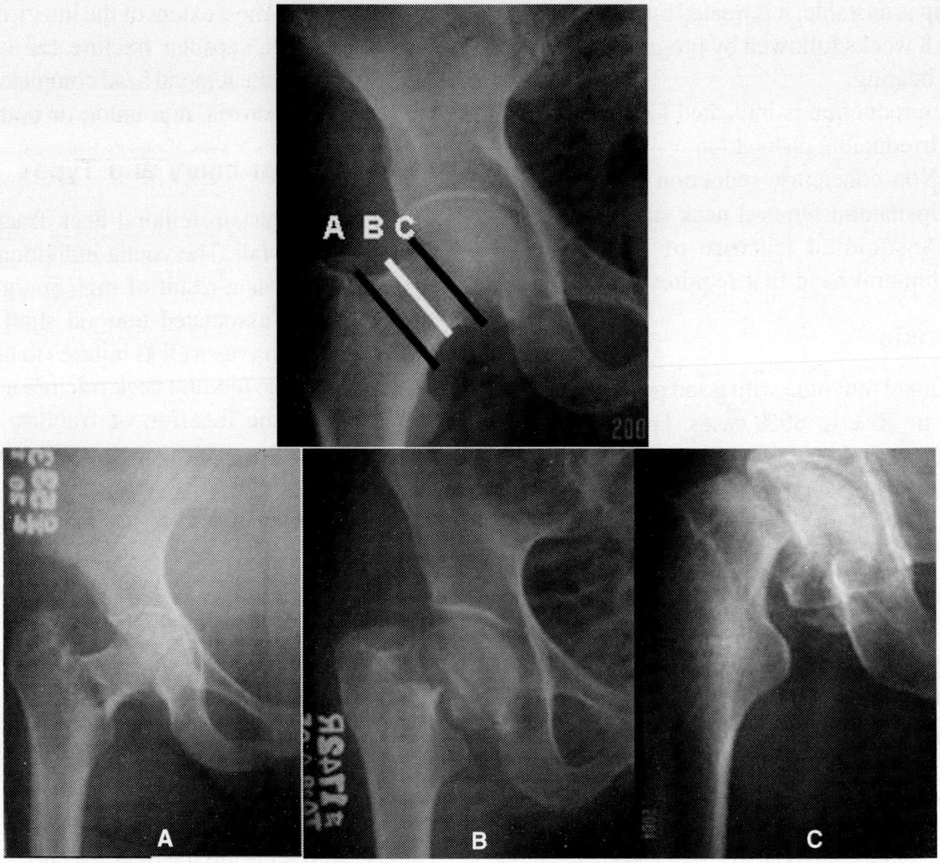

Fig. 10.8: Fracture neck of femur—Types. (A) Basicervical, (B) Transcervical, and (C) Subcapital

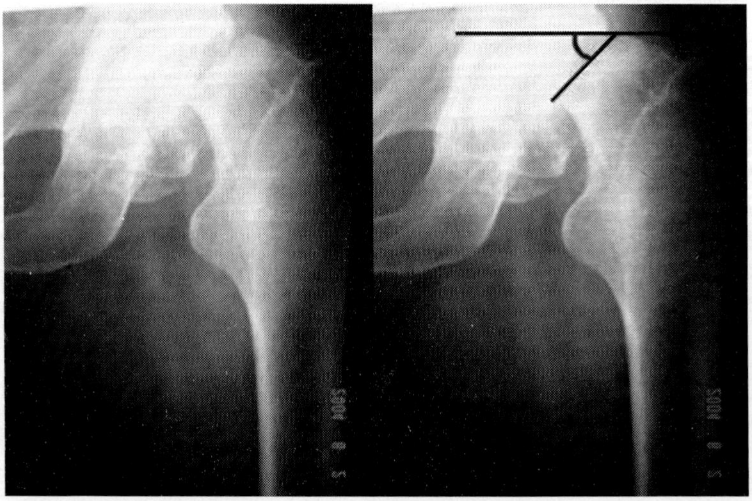

Fig. 10.9: Subcapital fracture neck of femur—Pauwel type II. This classification is important only for planning surgical treatment of non union of fracture neck of femur

Treatment

The goals of treatment are to minimize discomfort, prevent further damage, restore hip function and allow early mobilization by early anatomic reduction and stable internal fixation or by prosthetic replacement.

Non operative treatment is recommended only in patients who are unfit for operative treatment (medically or due to local condition of skin as infection, bed sore etc.).

Impacted or undisplaced fractures are treated with internal fixation with three cancellous screws.

Displaced fracture are treated according to the age of the patient (Fig. 10.10).

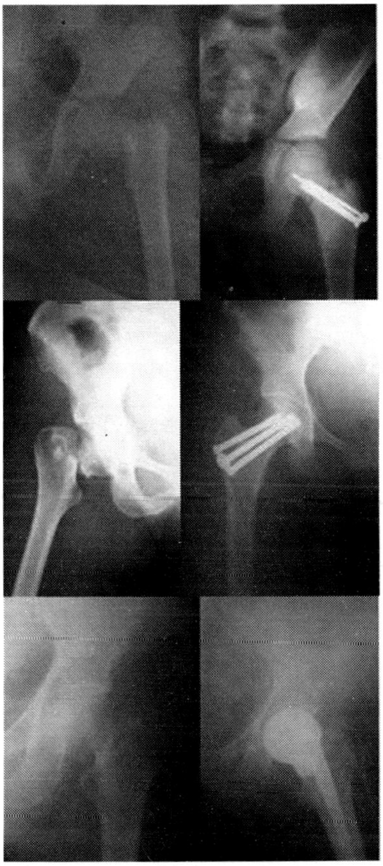

Fig. 10.10: Preferable treatment of fracture neck femur in (Top) children; (Middle) adult; and, (Bottom) old patients

Children are treated by closed reduction followed by fixation with 3 parallel Moore's or Knowles' pins. In children, the fracture may also be reduced by closed methods and immobilized in 1½ hip spica (Whitman's Spica).

Young patients are treated by urgent closed/ open (if closed reduction fails) reduction and internal fixation with 3 parallel cancellous screws.

Elderly patients with good bone density and high functional demands are treated by closed/open reduction and internal fixation.

Elderly patients with poor bone density and low functional demands are treated by hemiarthroplasty. Usually bipolar arthroplasty is performed for community ambulators while Austin Moore or Thompson prosthesis is inserted for patients who mainly remain indoors.

Patients with preexistent arthritic changes in acetabulum are treated by total hip replacement.

Complications

Non union (Fig. 10.11): Occurs because proximal fragment is small and osteoporotic, hence difficult to control and fix. Also, fracture hematoma is washed away by synovial fluid as the fracture is intra-articular. Young patients with non union are treated by muscle pedicle graft or proximal femoral osteotomy and bone grafting. Elderly patients with non union are treated by arthroplasty.

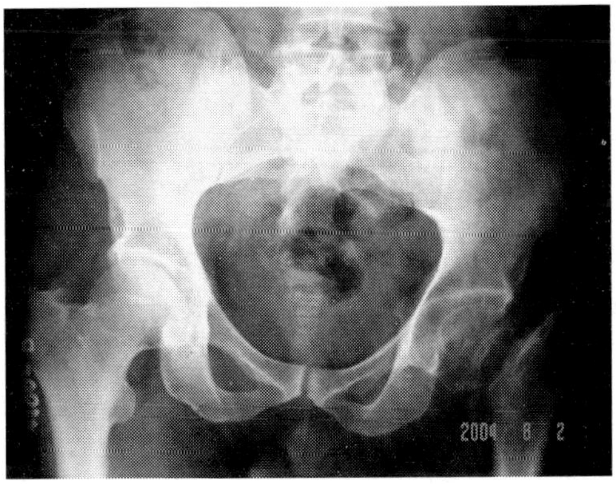

Fig. 10.11: Non union fracture neck of femur (L). Note the gap at the non union and osteoporosis of head fragment

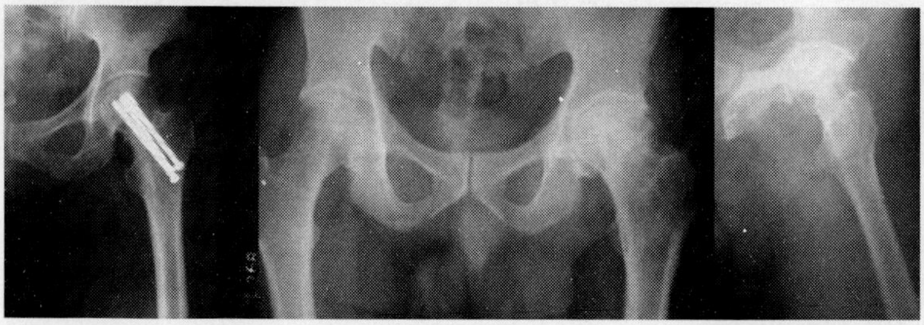

Fig. 10.12: Avascular necrosis of the femoral head following fracture neck of femur fixed with screws. Note the tracts of screws and increased density of the head. Also note that the fracture may sometimes unite in spite of avascular necrosis

Avascular Necrosis

Avascular necrosis leads to collapse of femoral head (Fig. 10.12). Young patients are preferably treated by arthrodesis while elderly are treated by arthroplasty.

Thromboembolism

Thromboembolism is common following hip fractures and surgery for hip fractures and thromboprophylaxis (with aspirin or Low Molecular Weight Heparin) should be used in all patients with hip fractures.

Fracture of Greater/Lesser Trochanter

Greater trochanter gives attachment to gluteus medius and minimus while iliopsoas attaches to lesser trochanter and these muscle attachments can avulse the respective trochanter. Greater trochanter fractures (Fig. 10.13) can also occur by direct impact as fall on the side. Minimally displaced greater trochanter fractures and isolated lesser trochanter fractures are ignored and treated with weight bearing as tolerated. Greater trochanter fractures displaced more than 1 cm are treated by fixation using screws or tension band wiring.

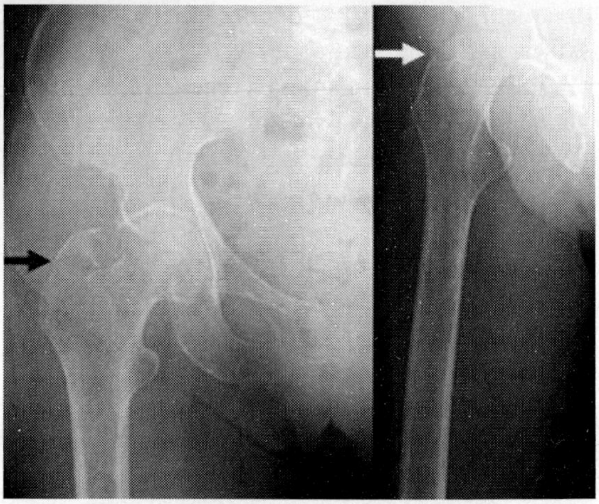

Fig. 10.13: Fracture of greater trochanter (arrow)

Intertrochanteric Fractures

Intertrochanteric fractures are extra capsular fractures and occur in older population than intra capsular fractures. These fractures are less difficult to treat than intracapsular fractures because of three reasons, namely:

a. Proximal fragment is larger and less mobile
b. The surface area of the fracture available for union is larger and consists of good cancellous bone, and,
c. The blood supply of the proximal fragment is not impaired and avascular necrosis is rare.

Mechanism of Injury and Types

The most common mechanism is direct injury by fall on the greater trochanter. Rarely indirect injury may lead to fracture by muscle forces transmitted to the intertrochanteric area.

The intertrochanteric fractures may be displaced or undisplaced. Displaced fractures are further differentiated by the direction and extent of the fracture line. The intertrochanteric fractures are also classified as stable or unstable depending on comminution and direction of fractures lines.

Clinical Features

Patient typically presents with inability to ambulate following a fall. The affected lower extremity is short and externally rotated (more so than

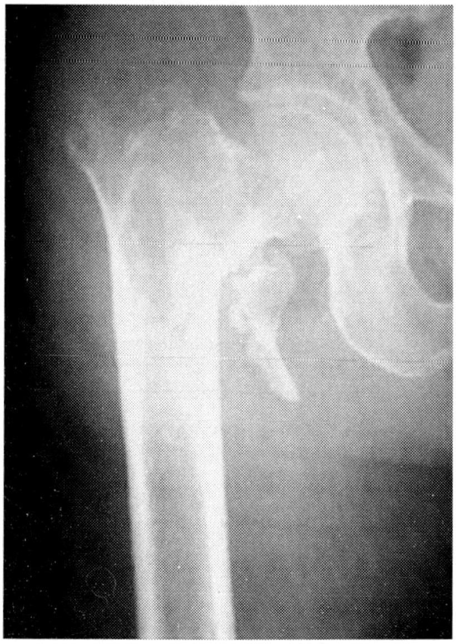

Fig. 10.14: Intertrochanteric fracture right femur

intracapsular fractures). There may be bruising, swelling and ecchymosis around the greater trochanter. Range of motion is painful with variable crepitus. Associated fractures of distal radius, proximal humerus, ribs and spine should be looked for. These patients often have medical comorbidities which should be looked for and managed.

X-rays

Anteroposterior view of the pelvis and hip (in internal rotation) and a cross table lateral view should be obtained. X-rays show the fracture line(s), displacements and degree of comminution (Fig. 10.14).

Treatment

Goal of treatment is to restore hip function and allow early mobilization by early anatomical reduction and stable internal fixation.

Non operative treatment is indicated only for those patients who were non ambulant before injury (due to dementia or other morbidities) or those who are at extreme medical risk for surgery. In these cases shortening and deformity (coxa vara) due to malunion are accepted.

Operative Treatment

The most common treatment is closed reduction and dynamic hip screw (or sliding hip screw)—DHS fixation of the fracture (Fig. 10.15). The implant is available in 130 to 150 degrees plate angles. The implant provides compression forces across the fracture and allows gradual controlled collapse and avoids implant failure.

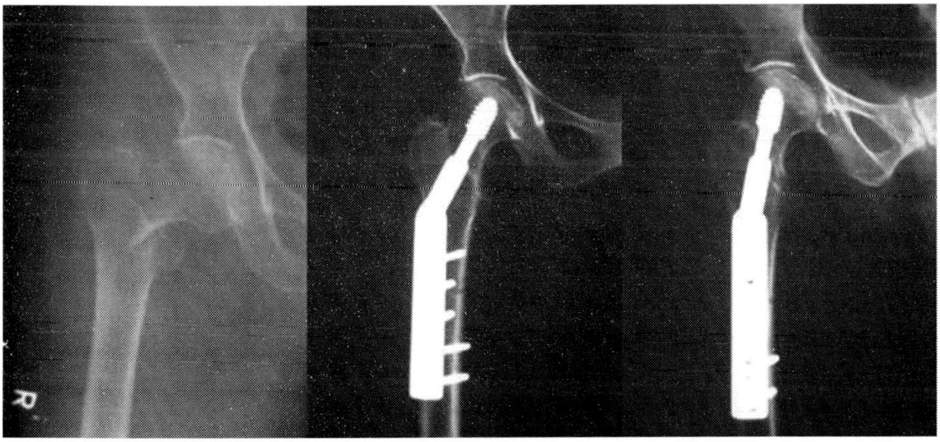

Fig. 10.15: Intertrochanteric fracture right femur fixed with Dynamic Hip Screw and barrel plate

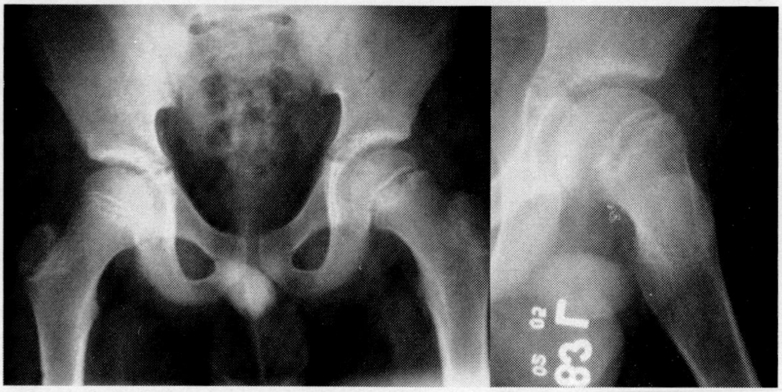

Fig. 10.16: Slipped capital femoral epiphysis. Note that the epiphysis slips inferiorly and posteriorly

Intra medullary hip screws (e.g. Gamma nail, Proximal Femoral Nail-PFN) have feature of sliding hip screw and intra medullary nail. These devices have not demonstrated any clinical advantage over DHS.

Rarely, a prosthetic replacement may be used for comminuted intertrochanteric fracture or when previous attempt at internal fixation has failed.

Following surgery the patients are mobilized non weight bearing with crutches for 6 to 8 weeks followed by protected partial weight bearing for another 4 to 6 weeks.

Complications

1. *Malunion* with varus of proximal fragment (coxa vara) is seen with conservative treatment or due to inability to achieve or maintain reduction. Coxa vara leads to shortening and lurch due to gluteus medius insufficiency.
2. *Nonunion* is seen following operative treatment in about 2% cases. Treatment consists of repeat fixation with valgus osteotomy and bone grafting or prosthetic replacement.
3. Malrotation deformity occurs due to fixation in internal rotation of distal fragment in unstable fracture patterns treated operatively.

Slipped Capital Femoral Epiphysis

The slipped capital femoral epiphysis in children can be traumatic (when it is anatomical equivalent of intra capsular fracture neck of femur) or atraumatic (when it occurs in adolescents due to hormonal/endocrine abnormalities).

When it occurs in the absence of trauma during the growth spurt, it is commoner in boys. The condition is often bilateral. The epiphysis slips posteriorly and inferiorly (Fig. 10.16) and the limb adopts a posture of adduction and internal rotation. Opposite hip should always be examined.

A slipped epiphysis is often followed by avascular necrosis and early osteoarthritis or chrondrolysis which leads to a stiff and painful hip with loss of joint space on X-rays.

Treatment

Treatment of slight or moderate displacement is in situ fixation with pins to prevent further slip.

Forceful manipulation can cause avascular necrosis and should be avoided.

Gross displacements are usually irreducible, especially when long standing and are treated by osteotomy when the growth is complete.

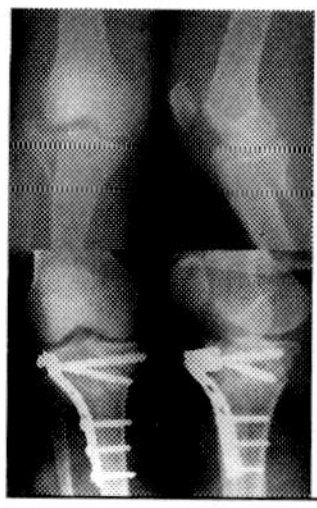

11

Injuries of Thigh and Knee

Femoral shaft, Subtrochanteric, Supracondylar, Femoral condyles, Tibial plateau, Patella, Knee dislocation, Patella dislocation, Knee ligaments, Menisci

FEMORAL SHAFT FRACTURES

Femoral shaft fracture is defined as a fracture of diaphysis occurring between 5 cm distal to lesser trochanter and 6 cm proximal to adductor tubercle.

Femoral shaft is a strong bone with an excellent blood supply and therefore good healing potential. Considerable violence is needed to fracture femoral shaft in young patients. Associated injuries are therefore, common and may be present in 5% to 15% cases. Patients often present with polytrauma including spine, pelvis and ipsilateral lower extremity injuries. Nearly 50% patients with closed femoral shaft fractures have ligamentous and meniscal injuries of the ipsilateral knee. Posterior dislocation of hip or femoral neck fractures may be associated.

The extensive musculature surrounding the femoral shaft is the cause of deformity of the thigh after a fracture:

- Lateral muscles inserting on greater trochanter (Abductors: gluteus medius and minimus) abduct the proximal femur after sub trochanteric fractures and proximal shaft fractures (*Caution:* Adducted proximal fragment here suggests associated posterior dislocation of ipsilateral hip!).
- Muscles inserting on lesser trochanter (Ilio-psoas) flex and externally rotate the proximal fragment in femoral shaft fractures.
- Adductors span most shaft fractures and exert traction on distal fragment (through their attachment on adductor tubercle) causing varus deformity in mid shaft fractures.
- Lateral thigh muscles and fascia lata resist varus forces of adductors and act as tension band.
- Gastrocnemius acts on distal shaft fractures and supracondylar fractures by angulating the distal fragment into flexion.

Fractures of the femoral shaft should be managed keeping the following cardinal principles in mind:

1. Intravenous access should be established and blood sent for haemoglobin estimation, grouping and cross matching in **all cases.** I.V. fluids should be infused and blood arranged.
2. X-ray pelvis with both hips and X-rays of the ipsilateral knee must be taken in **all cases.**
3. Associated injuries to other systems (skull, chest, abdomen) should be ruled out.
4. Patients should be placed in splints (preferably traction splints) to prevent muscle damage from jagged bone ends and to reduce the risk of fat embolism.

Mechanism of Injury and Types

Femoral shaft fractures in adults are almost always the result of high energy trauma such as motor vehicle accidents, gunshot injuries or falls from height. Any femoral fracture that occurs with trivial trauma should raise the suspicion of pathological fracture.

Femoral shaft fractures can be closed or open, located in proximal third, mid third or lower one third, can be transverse, oblique or spiral and can also be classified depending on the degree of comminution.

Clinical Features

Associated injuries must be considered in patients with suspected femoral shaft fracture and initial full trauma survey for associated injuries and resuscitation should precede detailed local examination unless a compound injury with active bleeding from the wound is present.

On local examination, the diagnosis of the femoral shaft fracture is obvious with the patient presenting with pain, inability to walk, gross swelling and deformity and shortening of the extremity. A careful neurovascular examination is essential. An expanding hematoma, absent or diminishing pulse and progressive neurologic signs in the presence of closed fracture suggest arterial injury. Ipsilateral limb injuries are common and should be looked for.

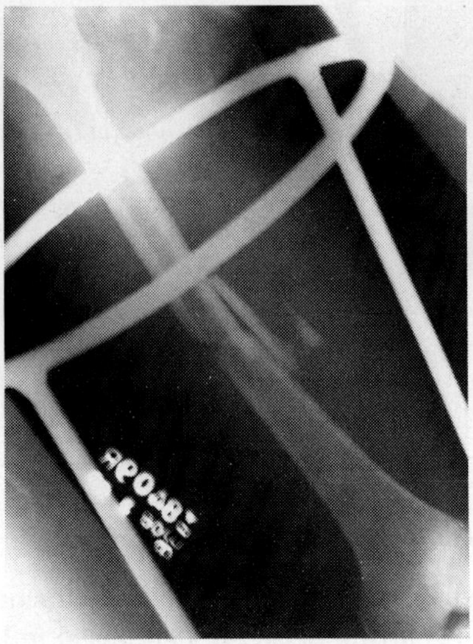

Fig. 11.1: Comminuted fracture shaft of femur-Middle third. Note the Thomas splint used to splint the fracture in casualty

X-rays

Before X-rays, emergency treatment is given and includes realignment of the injured extremity using skeletal traction, parenteral analgesics and wound toilet and sterile dressing application in case of compound fracture.

Anteroposterior and lateral views of the femur, hip and knee are obtained. An anteroposterior view of pelvis including both hips should also be obtained. Femoral neck should be carefully evaluated for fracture.

The femur X-rays should be evaluated for fracture pattern (spiral, oblique, transverse), complexity (simple, comminuted) and location (proximal, middle, distal third) (Fig. 11.1).

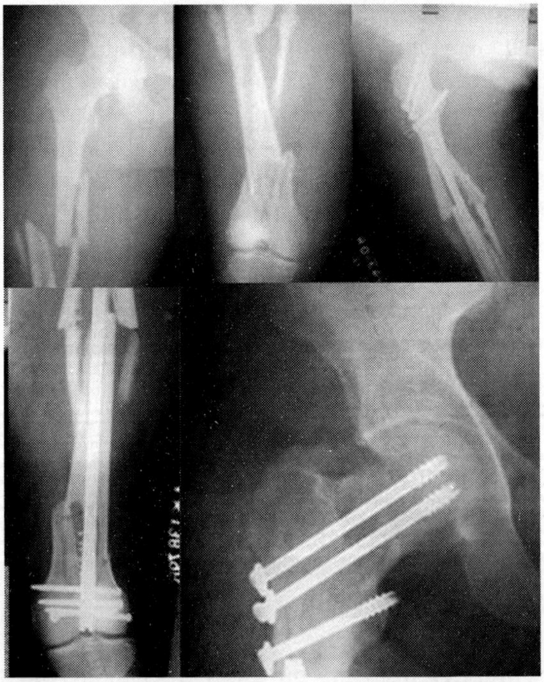

Fig. 11.2: (Top) Comminuted fracture of shaft femur associated with fracture neck femur; (Bottom) Treatment by intramedullary locking nail and AO screws (for femoral neck fracture)

Associated Injuries

Injuries associated with femoral shaft fracture include:

1. Ipsilateral femoral shaft and femoral neck fracture (Fig. 11.2).
2. Floating knee (ipsilateral femoral and tibial fractures) (Fig. 11.3).
3. Knee injuries: Patella fracture, knee ligament injuries

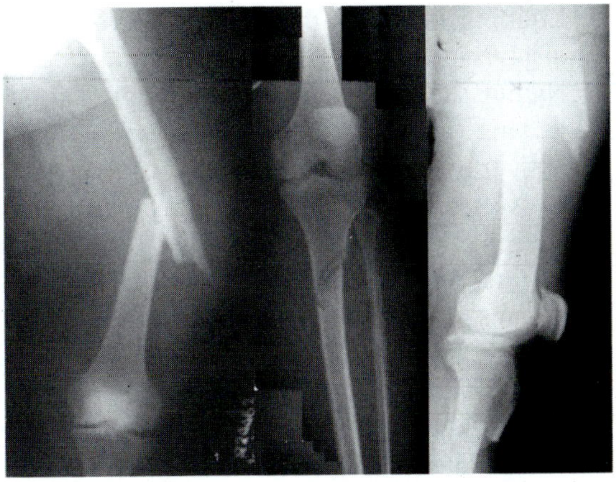

Fig. 11.3: Floating knee. Note the ipsilateral femoral shaft and proximal tibial fractures

4. Dislocation of ipsilateral hip
5. Fat embolism
6. Neurovascular injuries

Treatment

Fractures of the femoral shaft heal with immobilization using traction and casting but non operative methods require long hospitalization stays and the results are unpredictable. Malunion and knee stiffness are common if the non operative treatment is chosen for definitive treatment.

Non Operative Treatment

Skin traction is used for definitive fracture treatment only in young children. Bryant's or Gallow's traction (Fig. 4.5) is used for infants and suspends the child vertically through skin traction with the buttocks just lifted off the bed. Body weight of the child acts as counter traction force in these cases. In adults skin traction is used only for emergency fracture immobilization for patient comfort and to facilitate transport. Problems with skin traction are slippage and skin necrosis.

Skeletal traction (Fig. 11.4) is used today for early fracture care before definitive surgery but it is also indicated for the patients who are unfit for surgery. Skeletal traction aims to restore the femoral length and limit rotational and angular deformities. Problems associated with skeletal traction include pin tract infection, knee stiffness, shortening of limb, prolonged hospitalization, chest infection, urinary tract infection, decubitus ulcers and malunion.

Cast brace is an external support device that permits progressive weight bearing by circumferential support of the soft tissues thereby partially unloading the fracture. It is used after a period of skeletal traction. Healing occurs by 12 to 14 weeks. It is particularly useful for distal third

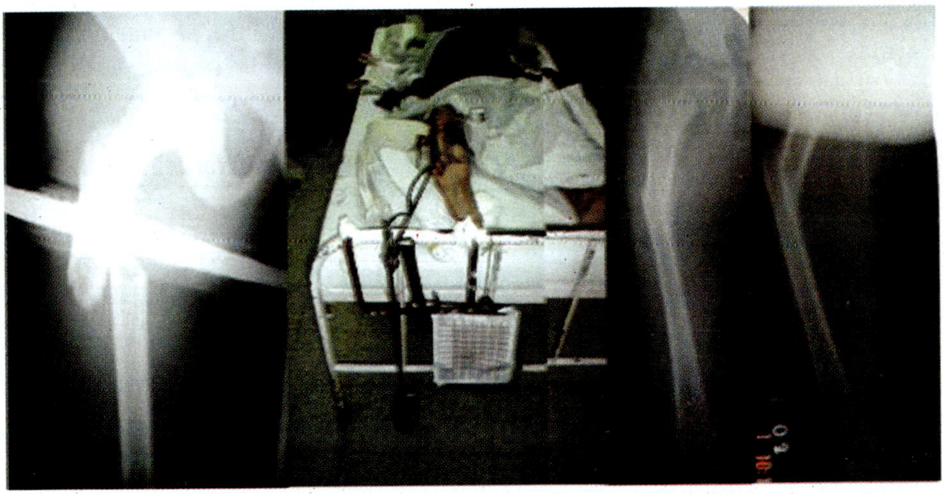

Fig. 11.4: Non operative treatment of femoral shaft fracture by skeletal traction. Note that malunion may occur as a complication of this method

and comminuted fractures. Problems associated with cast brace include loss of reduction and malunion.

Operative Treatment

Intra Medullary Nailing

An intramedullary nail is the treatment of choice for most femoral shaft fractures. The present generation of *locked intramedullary nails* have the following features that make them suitable for fixation of femoral shaft fractures (Fig. 11.5).

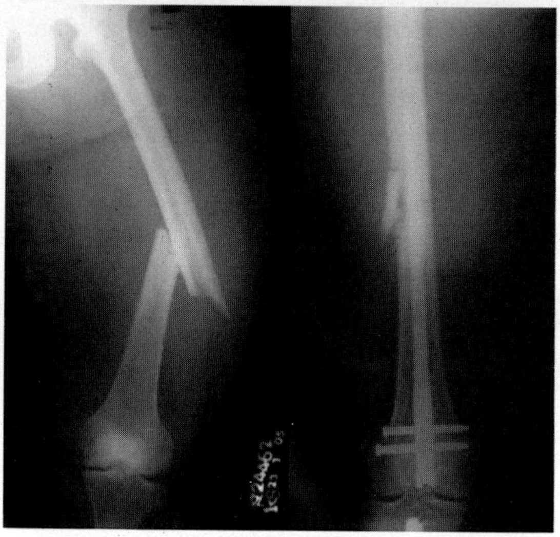

Fig. 11.5: Comminuted fracture shaft of femur treated by locked intramedullary nailing

1. Nail is a load-sharing device (compared to compression plate which is load-bearing device).
2. Can be inserted "closed" i.e. without opening the fracture site. Entry into the femoral medullary canal can be made through greater trochanter (antegrade) or through knee joint (retrograde). Less extensive exposure and preservation of fracture hematoma and soft tissue attachments expedite union.
3. Less dissection leads to reduced chance of infection, quadriceps scarring and knee stiffness.
4. Nailing allows early functional use of extremity.
5. Locking provides the control of rotational displacements.
6. Nailing can maintain length of femur by "static" locking (locking at both ends of nail-securing both fragments) in comminuted fractures. In transverse fractures with anatomical reduction, "dynamic" locking (locking only in the shorter fragment) provides compression at fracture site by muscle action and expedites union.

Interlocking nails, however, have the problems of technical difficulty in achieving closed reduction (as in cases with soft tissues interposition), need for image intersifier and radiation exposure to the surgeon as well as patient.

Antegrade nailing cannot be done in skeletally immature patients with open physes for the risk of damage to growth plate.

Kuntscher's nails are no more popular as they provide poor rotational stability. They, however, are still useful if image intensifier is not available or if patient cannot afford expensive interlocking nails.

Flexible intramedullary nails include Enders nails and rush pins but these offer poor rotational stability and results do not match those of locked nails.

Compression Plating

Femoral shaft fractures are treated by plating in skeletally immature patients and for stabilization of femoral shaft fractures associated with fractures of femoral neck (Fig. 11.6). Complications of plating include higher rates of infection (compared to nailing), loss of fixation, nonunion and refractures.

External Fixation

External fixation is indicated for open (compound) fractures. Fixator provides excellent bony fixation and wound access and allows early mobilization (Fig. 11.7). It may also serve as a temporary method of stabilization in patients who are too medically unstable to allow definitive intramedullary nailing.

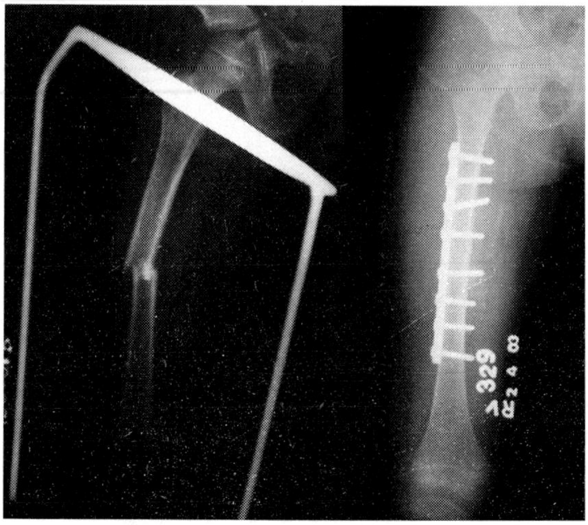

Fig. 11.6: Fracture shaft femur treated by plating in a child

Problems of external fixators include distraction of fracture, pin tract infection, pin loosening, knee stiffness and increased incidence of delayed union and non union.

Following fixation of femoral fractures patient is kept non weight bearing for 12-16 weeks. Following interlocking nailing, full weight bearing is begun when the fracture callus involving three cortices is seen.

Complications

a. Complications due to injury
   1. Neurovascular injuries: are uncommon due to large muscular envelope around femur. Vascular injury may occur due to tethering of the femoral artery at the adductor hiatus.

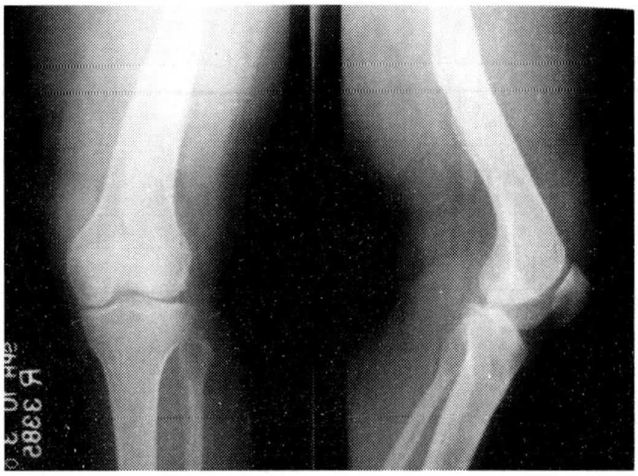

Fig. 11.8: Malunited femoral shaft fracture

   2. Fat embolism syndrome
b. Complication of union
   1. Non union, delayed union
   2. Malunion, usually varus, internal rotation and/or shortening (Fig. 11.8)
   3. Refracture following healing
c. Complications of treatment
   1. Infection
   2. Failure of fixation (breakage of implants)
   3. Knee stiffness
   4. Peroneal nerve palsy (due to traction)

OTHER INJURIES OF THIGH REGION

Subtrochanteric Fractures

Subtrochanteric fractures are fractures occurring within 5 cm of lesser trochanter (extending from inferior portion of lesser trochanter distally to the isthmus of the femoral shaft). These fractures have bimodal distribution.

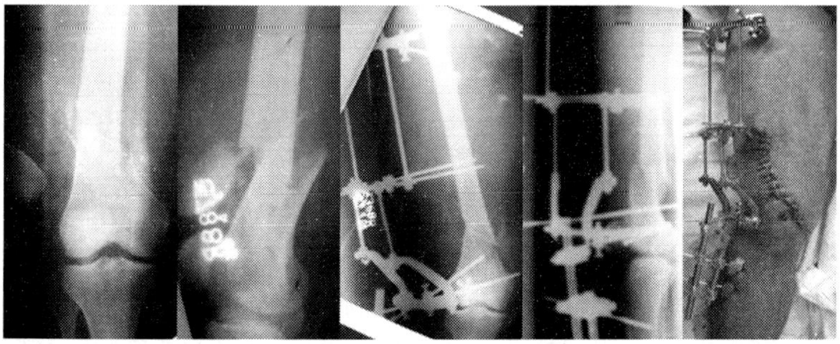

Fig. 11.7: Compound facture shaft of femur managed by external fixator

These are caused by high energy injuries in young adults and minor fall in elderly. Young patients often have associated injuries. Significant internal bleeding can occur in thigh. The deforming forces include gluteus medius which abducts the proximal fragment, external rotators (externally rotate) and iliopsoas (flexes proximal fragment). The distal fragment is pulled proximally and into varus by adductors. Non operative treatment (skeletal traction in 90°-90° position followed by spica cast or cast bracing) is reserved for patients unfit for surgery and results in increased morbidity and mortality. Operative treatment is by interlocking nails (when trochanters are intact) (Fig. 11.9), sliding hip screw, special (95° fixed angle) plates, intramedullary hip screw devices (like Zickel nail, gamma nail) or Enders nails. Common complications include malunion and non union.

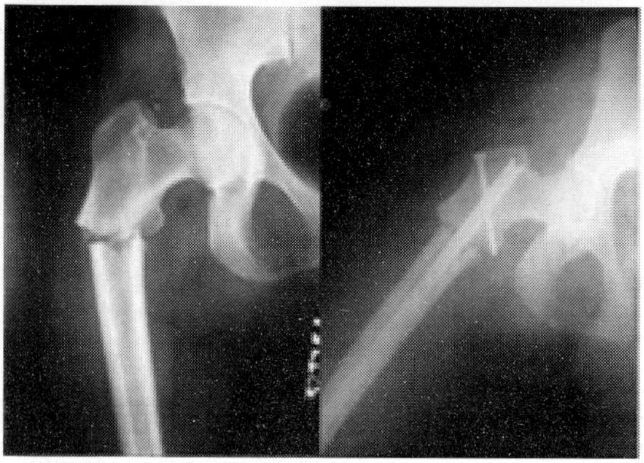

Fig. 11.9: Subtrochanteric fracture right femur treated by interlocking nail

Distal Femur (Supracondylar) Fractures

These fractures also have bimodal distribution. In young patients these are caused by high energy trauma while in elderly they occur following trivial falls. Deforming forces from muscular attachments cause characteristic displacements. Gastrocnemius flexes distal fragment and causes posterior angulation and displacement. Quadriceps and hamstrings cause shortening of extremity. Anteroposterior and lateral X-ray of lower femur including knee should be obtained (Fig. 11.10). Oblique views or CT scan may be needed to rule out extension of fracture lines into the knee joint. Non operative treatment is reserved for undisplaced, impacted, severely osteoporotic fractures or when the patient is unfit for surgery.

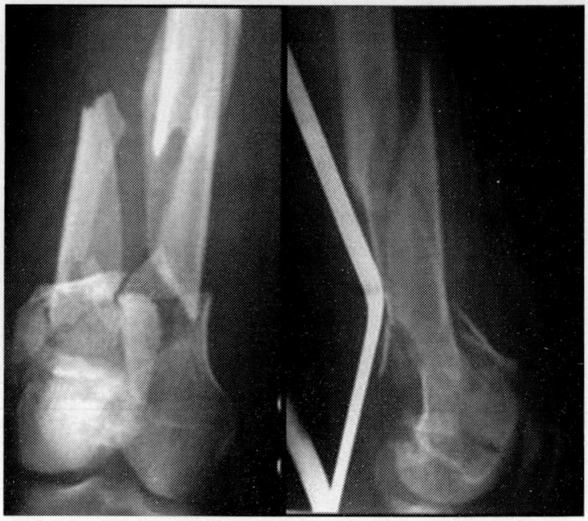

Fig. 11.10: Comminuted supracondylar fracture of femur with intercondylar extension

Operative treatment is indicated for open fractures, associated displaced intraarticular fractures, associated neurovascular injuries, pathological fractures and floating knee (associated tibia fracture in same extremity). Implants used for fixation include Dynamic condylar screw, 95° condylar blade plate, Supracondylar (locked retrograde IM) nails and external fixator. Complications include malunion, non union, knee stiffness and infection.

Wagon Wheel Injury is the distal femoral epiphyseal injury seen in adolescents when they try to climb aboard a wagon while chasing it. Treatment is anatomical reduction and stabilization by crossed K wires (Fig. 11.11).

Injuries Around Knee

The knee is vulnerable to injury during sports, dashboard injuries or falls. Knee is an inherently unstable joint given the asymmetry between the

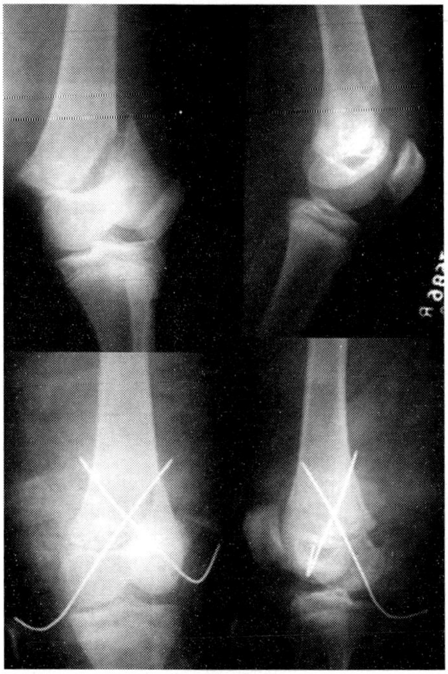

Fig. 11.11: Wagon Wheel Injury. (Top) Epiphyseal injury distal femur. (Bottom) Treated by reduction and cross K-wire fixation

shape of femoral and tibial condyles and knee relies largely on the supporting soft tissues for stability. Medial and lateral collateral ligaments resist valgus and varus forces respectively. Anterior cruciate ligament keeps the tibia from translating anteriorly in relation to the distal femur and the posterior cruciate ligament keeps the tibia from displacing excessively backwards. Medial and lateral menisci improve congruency between the femoral and tibial condyles, increase the surface area of articulation and act as shock absorbers. Neurovascular structures are intimately related to the posterior aspect of the knee and are prone to injury. Careful assessment, clinically as well as radiologically, is required for accurate diagnosis of knee injuries to treat them adequately. Examination under anaesthesia (for ligament injuries), CT scan (for intraarticular fractures) and MRI (for ligaments, menisci) are often useful. Arthroscopy is being increasingly used to accurately identify and treat the various traumatic and non traumatic pathologies within the knee.

FRACTURES OF DISTAL FEMUR AND PROXIMAL TIBIA

Femoral Condylar Fractures

Fractures entering the intercondylar notch of femur can break one or both femoral condyles away from the femoral shaft. The fractures can be undisplaced or displaced. Clinically these fractures present with swelling of the knee and hemarthrosis with or without significant deformity. Patient is unable to bear weight on the injured extremity. Careful neurovascular examination must be performed in all cases. Anteroposterior and lateral radiographs of the knee suffice though oblique views and CT scan may be required sometimes for evaluating intraarticular displacement. Treatment depends on degree of displacement. Goal of treatment is anatomic fracture reduction, stable internal fixation and early joint motion to prevent stiffness and degenerative osteoarthritis. Undisplaced fractures and fractures in elderly who are infirm are treated in traction for 4 weeks followed by plaster immobilization for 8 weeks.

Displaced fractures are operated and open reduction and internal fixation is done. Fractures of a single condyle are treated by fixation using screws (Fig. 11.12). Fractures of both condyles are treated initially by fixing the condyles together using screws, converting intercondylar fracture into supracondylar fracture, which is then fixed to diaphysis using 95° angle blade plate, Dynamic condylar screw or supracondylar nail. Complications include stiffness of the knee, injury to neurovascular structures, avascular necrosis of condylar fragments, malunion with varus/valgus deformity and secondary osteoarthritis.

Tibial Plateau Fractures

The tibial plateau fractures are caused by high-velocity trauma in young adults and following trivial fall in the elderly osteoporotic men. The tibial

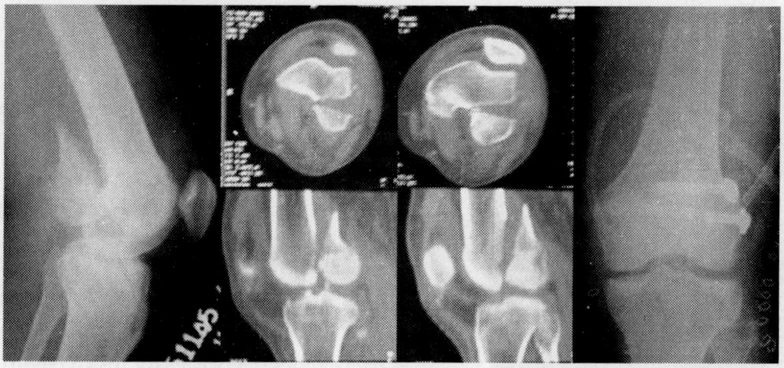

Fig. 11.12: Fractures of single condyle of femur (left) are well evaluated by CT scan (middle), treatment is by screw fixation (right)

fractures are classified according to the condyle (medial/lateral) involved and whether articular surface is split or depressed. If the knee is struck violently on the lateral side, the resultant valgus force on the knee can tear medial collateral ligament or cause fracture of the lateral tibial plateau (Bumper fracture). Patient presents with swelling of the knee, hemarthrosis, pain and inability to ambulate. Anteroposterior and lateral X-rays diagnose the fracture but oblique views and CT scan are required often to assess articular involvement and joint depression. Treatment aims to restore knee function by accurate reduction, stable internal fixation and early joint motion. Undisplaced fractures can be treated in long leg cast for 8-10 weeks. Patient is advised to ambulate non weight bearing with crutches. If a large fragment is split off, it is reduced and fixed with screws with or without supporting ("buttress") plate (Fig. 11.13). Large depressed fragments can be elevated to reconstitute articular surface. This leaves a large defect under the articular cartilage where cancellous bone was crushed. This cavity is filled with cancellous bone grafts taken from the iliac crest or by synthetic Calcium Phosphate cement. These fractures are now increasingly fixed by arthroscopy assisted techniques where arthroscopy is used to confirm the accuracy of articular surface reduction.

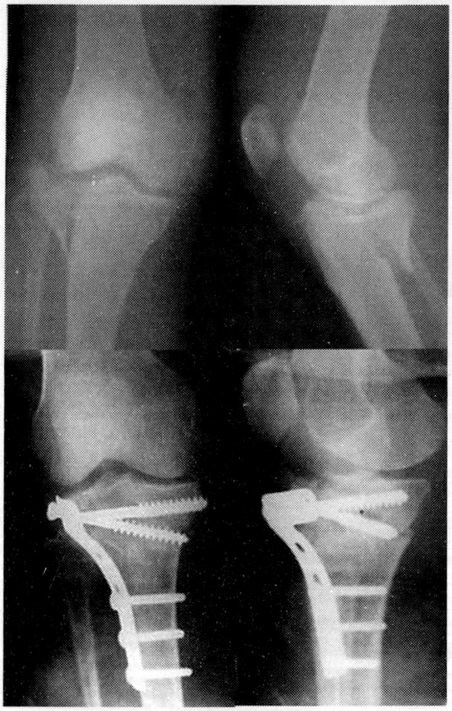

Fig. 11.13: (Top) Fracture of the lateral tibial condyle (Bottom) Treated with restoration of articular surface (by elevation and bone grafting) and buttress plating

Complications of tibial plateau fractures include injury to neuro vascular structures, malunion with varus/valgus deformity, associated injury to ligaments/menisci, secondary osteoarthritis of the knee and stiffness of knee.

Osteochondral Fractures

Osteochondral fragments may be sheared off by direct trauma or avulsed by indirect injury. Clinically these fractures present with hemarthrosis. Fracture fragment may be wholly cartilaginous and may not be detected on plain X-rays but hemarthrosis and fat from the cancellous bone which forms fat fluid level on lateral radiograph suggest the diagnosis. MRI and arthroscopy can confirm the diagnosis. If left untreated, the fragment may present later as a loose body. Treatment is arthroscopic removal of small fragments and reattachment of large fragments using special pins/headless screws.

DISRUPTION OF EXTENSOR MECHANISM

Extension at the knee is brought about by the action of an intact extensor mechanism which consists of quadriceps muscle (especially rectus femoris), quadriceps tendon, patella, patellar ligament alongwith patellar retinaculae (longitudinal extensions of the quadriceps tendon passing medial and lateral to patella and inserting directly on anterior tibia), and, tibial tuberosity. Disruption of extensor mechanism at any point interferes with knee extension. Thus rupture of rectus femoris, rupture of quadriceps tendon, fracture of patella with tear in patellar retinaculae, rupture of patellar ligament and avulsion of tibial tuberosity all interfere with knee extension (Fig. 11.14).

Fractures of the Patella

Patella is the largest sesamoid bone in the body. It forms a part of the extensor mechanism of the knee and functions to improve the lever arm of the extensor mechanism. Patella is prone to injury due to its subcutaneous location.

Mechanisms of Injury and Types

Classification of patellar fractures is based on the morphology of fracture which is determined by the mechanism of injury.

Direct Trauma due to fall on the knee or direct blow (as in dash board injury) on the knee gives rise to comminuted or stellate fracture. These fractures are generally undisplaced. Extensor mechanism is usually not disrupted.

Indirect Trauma occurs when there is violent contraction of quadriceps in a flexed knee as while trying to break a fall. It results in transverse fractures. These fractures are usually displaced and are associated with disruption of the extensor mechanism.

Clinical Features

Patient presents with history of direct blow to anterior knee or forced and rapid knee flexion against contracted quadriceps, anterior knee pain and an inability to extend the knee. Patient has pain, swelling and inability to walk. On examination, a gap may be palpable in patella and extension lag is present. Associated injuries (ipsilateral femoral shaft, distal femoral, proximal tibial fractures or posterior dislocation of hip) should be looked for.

X-rays

Patella is difficult to visualize on anteroposterior view but is well visualized on lateral X-ray. Articular

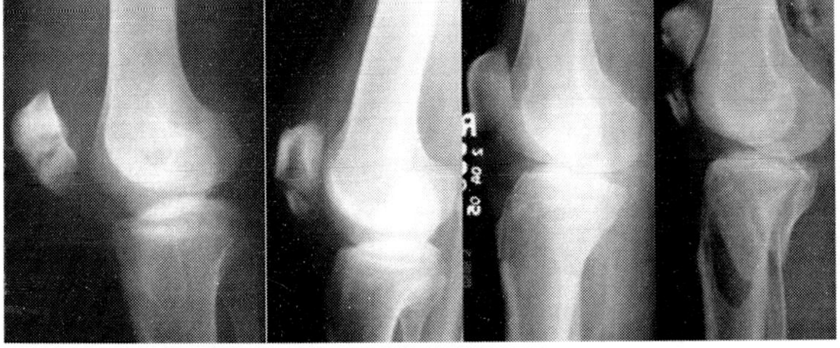

Fig. 11.14: (Extreme left): Transverse fracture patella (Second from left): Inferior pole fracture patella (Third from left): Tibial tuberosity avulsion (Extreme right): Associated proximal tibia fracture. Note that fracture patella may be associated with other major fractures in the region

step off and separation of fragments is assessed. Bilateral X-rays should be advised if there is smooth superolateral fragment suggesting bipartite patella which is a congenital variant and often bilateral and should not be confused with the fracture.

Treatment

Non operative treatment is indicated for undisplaced fractures where patient is actively able to extend the knee. A long leg cylinder cast is applied for 4 to 6 weeks. Patient is allowed to bear weight as tolerated.

Operative treatment is indicated for displaced patellar fractures with loss of extensor function. Goal of surgery is to preserve patellar function and restore anatomy of patellar articular surface. Multiple methods for fixation exist such as:

- Tension band wiring (circular or figure of 8) with parallel longitudinal Kirschner wires (Fig. 11.15).
- Circumferential wiring
- Cancellous lag screw fixation-alone or with tension band.

Retinacular disruption is repaired. Patient is encouraged to perform active assisted range of motion exercises for the knee and is allowed to progress to partial or full weight bearing by 6 weeks. However, in cases of comminuted fractures, where restoration of congruent articular surface is not possible, patellectomy (partial or total) has to be considered.

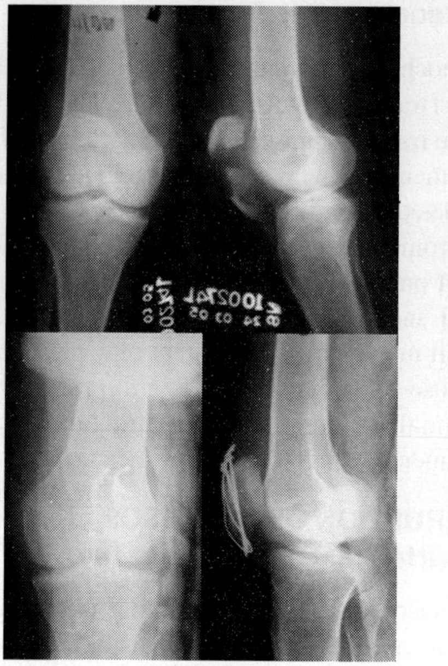

Fig. 11.15: (Top) Fracture patella treated by (Bottom) tension band wiring

Partial patellectomy is done when there is polar comminution (at proximal or distal pole) with a large salvageable fragment and achieving stable fixation or restoring articular surface is impossible (Fig. 11.16). The comminuted fragments are excised and quadriceps or patellar tendon is reattached to the remaining fragment close to its articular surface to prevent patellar tilt.

Total patellectomy is reserved for cases with extensive and severe comminution. Medial and

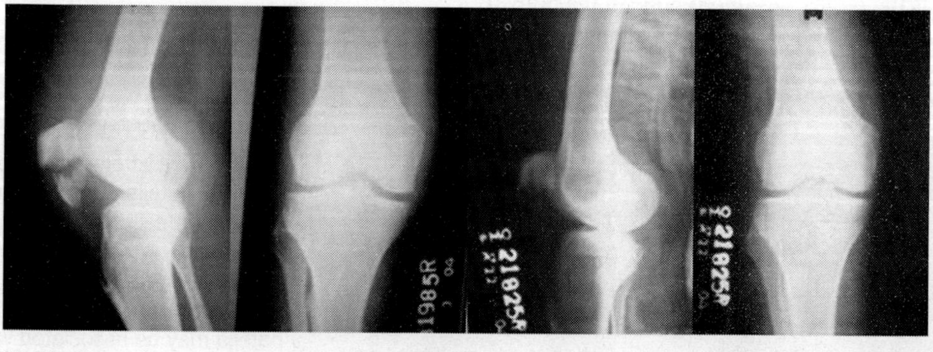

Fig. 11.16: Comminuted fracture of patella treated by partial (lower pole in this case) patellectomy

lateral retinaculae are repaired. The power of quadriceps, however, is reduced.

Postoperatively, the knee is immobilized in a long leg cast in extension for 3 to 6 weeks.

Complications of Patellar Fractures

1. Loss of range of motion (knee stiffness)
2. Post traumatic osteoarthritis
3. Infection following surgery
4. Loss of fixation
5. Pain due to hardware (tension band wiring)
6. Nonunion-rare (2%)
7. Refracture
8. Avascular necrosis of proximal fragment.

KNEE DISLOCATION

Knee dislocation is rare but can be limb threatening due to potential for injury to neurovascular structures present in the popliteal fossa. Complete separation of the tibia from the femur requires enough trauma to tear all the ligaments and the joint capsule. Knee dislocations are caused by high energy trauma such as motor vehicle accidents, dashboard injuries etc. Knee dislocation is classified based on the displacement of the proximal tibia relative to the distal femur and may be anterior (most common), posterior, lateral, medial or rotational. It may be a pure dislocation (Fig. 11.17A) or associated with a fracture (Fig. 11.17B). Clinically, patients present with gross knee distortion. Immediate reduction should be performed. Vascular (popliteal artery) injury is reported in 20-60% cases and may present as late as one week after injury due to late thrombosis related to intimal injury. Neurologic injury (Peroneal nerve) is present in 10-35% cases. Plain X-rays are diagnostic but since the condition is potentially limb threatening, immediate reduction of dislocation is recommended before X-rays. After reduction, X-rays can be taken to evaluate adequacy of reduction. Angiography is indicated in obvious or suspected thrombosis and vascular occlusion. MRI may be essential to assess extent of soft tissue injury.

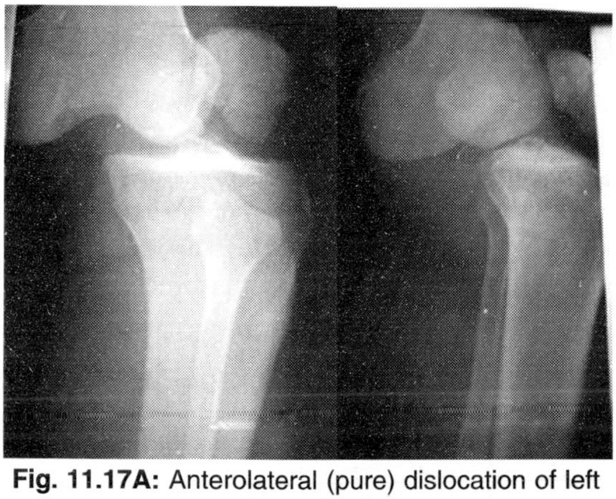

Fig. 11.17A: Anterolateral (pure) dislocation of left knee joint

Treatment is immediate reduction by traction and manipulation. Irreducible dislocations should be operated to achieve reduction. Vascular injuries require external fixation and vascular repair with reverse saphenous vein graft. Following reduction limb should be splinted in 20 to 30 degrees of flexion. Range of motion exercises are started after soft tissue healing (6 to 12 weeks).

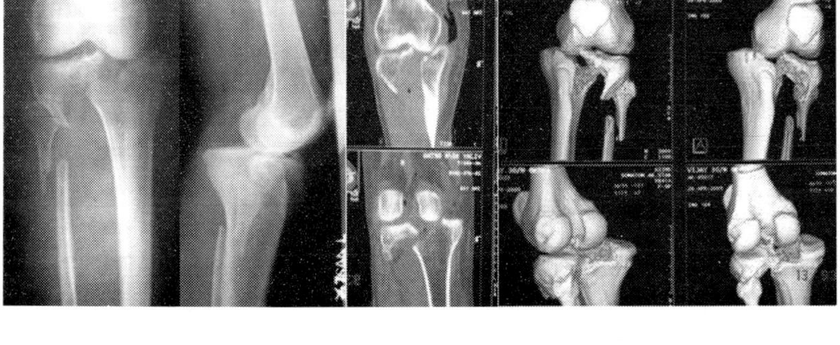

Fig. 11.17B: Fracture dislocation of right knee joint. (Left) plain X-rays. Note that both tibia and fibula are fractured. (Middle) CT scan, coronal cuts delineate the fracture line extending into the joint. (Right) 3D reconstruction provides additional information about the fragments and their displacements

Complications

1. Vascular compromise: may present acutely or after 24-72 hours
2. Compartment syndrome
3. Nerve injury-generally prognosis is poor
4. Knee stiffness-most common complication
5. Ligamentous laxity and instability.

Patellar Dislocation

Patellar dislocations (Fig. 11.18) are common in adolescent females and in patients with hypermobility and connective tissue disorders. Patella can dislocate during soccer, baseball, gymnastics, karate or dancing. Most common type of patella dislocation is lateral which is caused by a sharp twisting (internal rotation of femur on externally rotated tibia) movement of the knee in flexion. Patella sometimes reduces itself at once but if it remains dislocated, patient remembers seeing the knee cap on the outer aspect of the knee. On examination after a dislocation, knee is swollen due to hemarthrosis and there is tenderness on the medial side due to tear of medial structures. X-rays show hemarthrosis, sometimes a fat fluid level

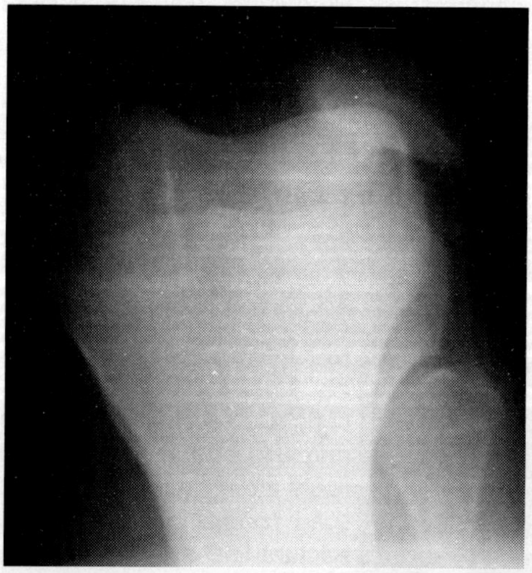

Fig. 11.18: Dislocation of patella. Note that dislocation is almost always lateral. The view shown (Skyline or sunrise) is the best view for patellofemoral joint pathologies

and rarely an osteochondral (chip) fracture fragment on medial side of patella.

Treatment is reduction and above knee cylinder cast in extension for 3 weeks followed by physiotherapy to regain flexion gradually over next 4 to 6 weeks.

Complications

1. Redislocation
2. Stiffness of knee
3. Patellofemoral pain.

The clinical syndrome of patellar dislocation has a spectrum.

1. Acute dislocation-as described above.
2. Recurrent dislocation-Repeated episodes of patellar dislocation
3. Habitual dislocation-dislocation of patella *every* time the patient flexes the knee.

Recurrent and habitual patellar dislocations are seen in association with shallow trochlear groove, small high riding patella, genu valgum, or high angle ('Q' angle) between the line of pull of Quadriceps tendon and patellar ligament. The patellofemoral instability is addressed by correction of all malalignment factors. Surgical options include lateral retinacular release, medial retinacular plication and proximal and/or distal patellar realignment procedures to alter the direction of pull of quadriceps mechanism.

Ligament Injuries at the Knee

Ligament injuries are common around knee and are often missed as they do not show on radiographs. As ligaments never heal soundly or regain their normal strength following injury, ligamentous injuries have more serious long term implications than fractures. Incomplete healing of the ligaments may give rise to long-term instability of the joint, with feeling of "giving way".

Injuries of Collateral Ligaments

Strains of the collateral ligaments are common after sporting injuries. Partial tears of ligaments are typically more painful than complete ruptures.

Strains are associated with an acute effusion in the knee joint and tenderness over the damaged ligament. Stressing the ligament causes pain, but the joint remains stable. Medial collateral ligament is injured by valgus stress while lateral collateral ligament is injured by varus stress.

In addition, valgus strain combined with rotational force at knee (external rotation) with flexion while weight bearing can cause Medial Collateral ligament tear, Anterior Cruciate Ligament (ACL) tear and medial meniscus injury—so called *O'Donogue or unhappy triad* seen in American footballers. Isolated lesions of the medial collateral ligament (MCL) and lateral collateral ligament (LCL) (Fig. 11.19) can usually heal well without operation and are treated in above knee cylinder cast in 10 degrees flexion for 6 weeks.

Lesions near femoral attachment can heal with the formation of a flake of new bone which can be seen radiographically. The site of injury may remain tender for several years. Tenderness associated with radiological signs of an old medial ligament injury is known as "Pellegrini-Steida disease".

Anterior Cruciate Ligament Injury

Anterior cruciate ligament (ACL) limits forward movement of tibia on femur and is often ruptured in sporting activities by a sharp twisting movement.

ACL tear is a common injury and accounts for 75% cases of acute hemarthrosis. Patient feels giving way, a break or "pop" in the knee at the time of injury and it is soon followed by swelling and muscle spasm.

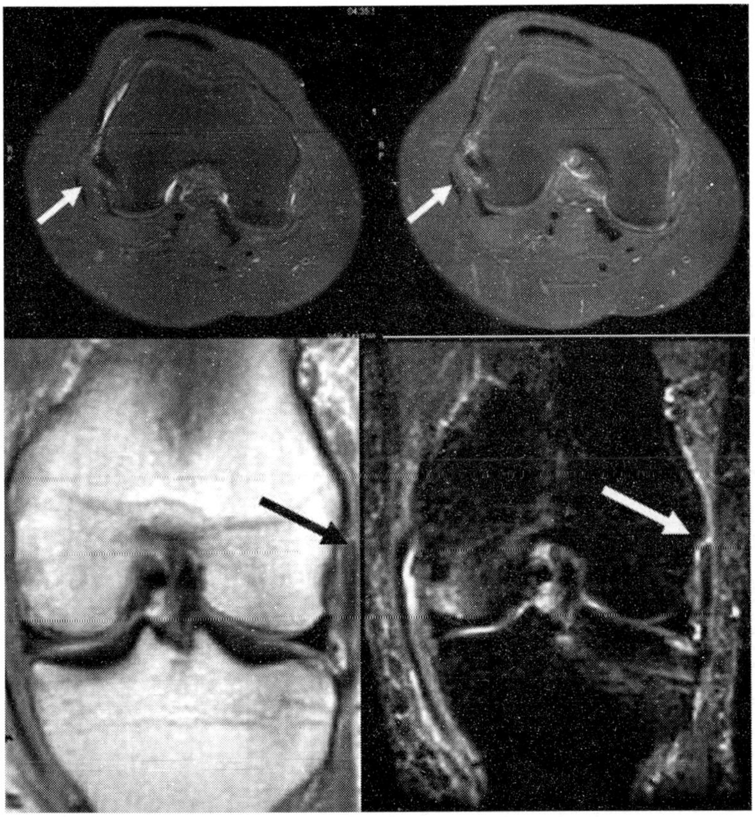

Fig. 11.19: (Top) Medial collateral ligament injury (short arrows); (Bottom) Lateral collateral ligament injury (long arrows)—MRI picture

Examination immediately after injury or subsequently under anaesthesia reveals a positive Lachman and Anterior Drawer test. X-ray are mostly normal except when bony avulsion has occurred (Fig. 11.20A). MRI is non invasive investigation and is diagnostic (Fig. 11.20B). ACL injury gives rise to instability though about one third patients achieve good result without surgery. In patients who pursue sporting activities and are high demand, operative treatment is undertaken. Effective repair of ligament is impossible and reconstruction of ligament using patellar tendon graft (Middle 1/3rd) or hamstring tendons is done. Bony avulsion of ACL is treated by fixation under arthroscopic control.

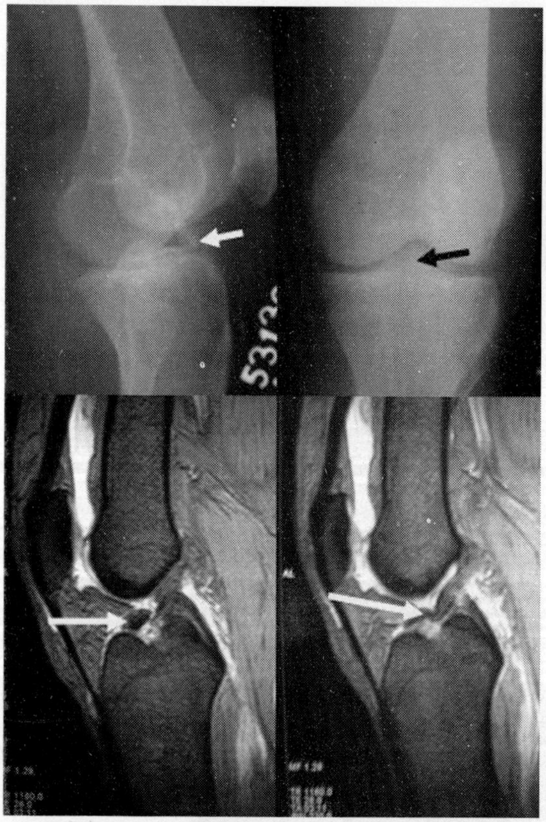

Fig. 11.20A: (Top) Avulsion of tibial spine seen on plain X-rays (short arrows); (Bottom) MRI shows avulsed fragment and buckling of ACL (long arrows)

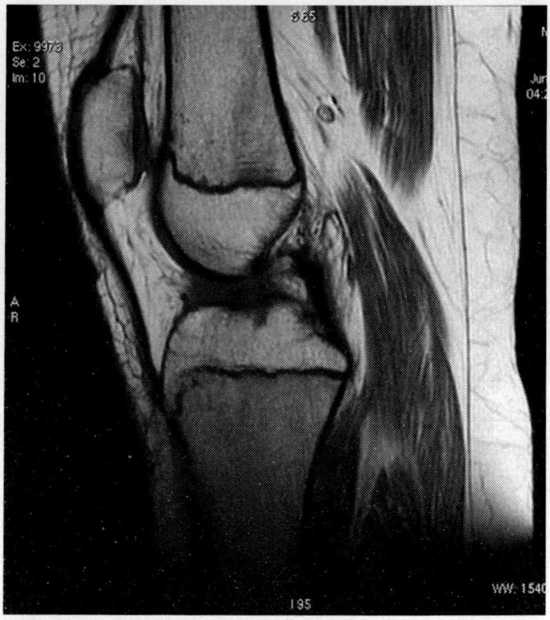

Fig. 11.20B: MRI picture of anterior cruciate ligament tear. Note that the normal ACL is absent. Also note the presence of PCL (Posterior cruciate ligament)

Posterior Cruciate Ligament (PCL)

A PCL can be torn by blow to anterior end of tibia when knee is flexed (as in dashboard injury) or by hyperextension. Examination reveals hemarthrosis and backward sag of tibia relative to femur (recurvatum). MRI is non invasive investigation and is diagnostic (Fig. 11.21). Most patients with isolated PCL rupture make excellent recovery without treatment and conservative treatment is adequate. Operative treatment is considered when there is a bony avulsion (which can be reattached to its bed) or any other associated ligament injury.

Meniscal Injury

Medial meniscus is "C" shaped structure attached at each end to intercondylar eminence and at its mid point to the deep medial capsular ligament. Lateral meniscus is "O" shaped and attached medially to intercondylar eminence. Medial meniscus is injured more commonly than lateral because (of):

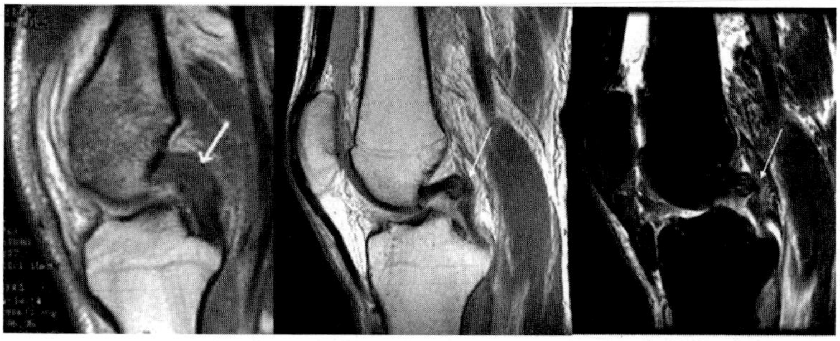

Fig. 11.21: MRI picture of posterior cruciate ligament tear (arrow)

- Its shape
- Its relative immobility (It is attached to the deep medial capsular ligament)
- Lateral meniscus has single medial attachment.
- Popliteus is attached to lateral meniscus and provides mobility to it thus preventing injury.

Menisci move posteriorly with flexion and anteriorly with extension.

Meniscal tears occur due to violent stretching or crushing force between femoral and tibial condyles during sudden rotary or extension-flexion injuries. Patients may present with repeated episodes of joint locking when a free segment of meniscus displaces into joint.

Meniscal injuries present with triad of joint line pain, swelling and locking. Several clinical signs are described which aim to trap the torn portion of meniscus between the femoral and tibial condyles (McMurray's test, Steinmann sign etc.). MRI is diagnostic (Fig. 11.22). Arthroscopy is diagnostic and therapeutic (Fig. 11.23).

Treatment of meniscal tear is according to symptoms. Acutely locked knee is reduced with the extremity hanging off the edge of the table and

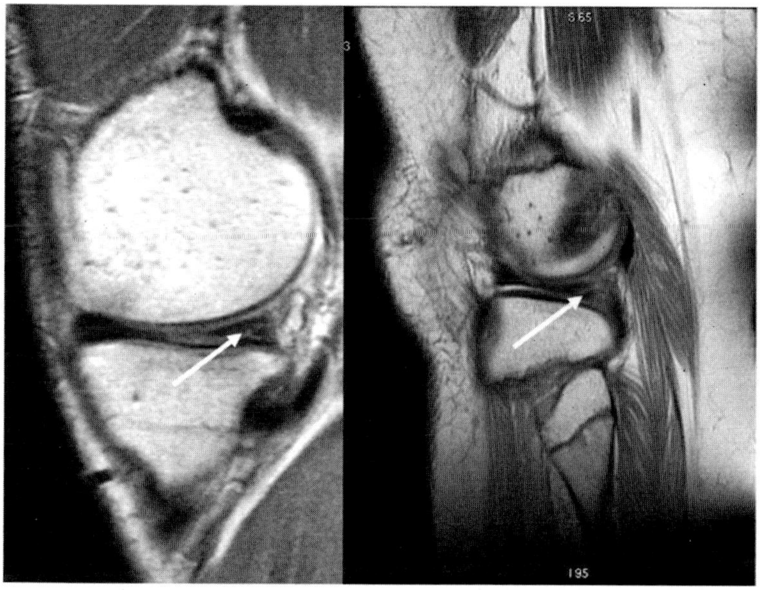

Fig. 11.22: Meniscal tears seen on MRI. (Left) Posterior horn tear of medial meniscus; (Right) Posterior horn tear of lateral meniscus

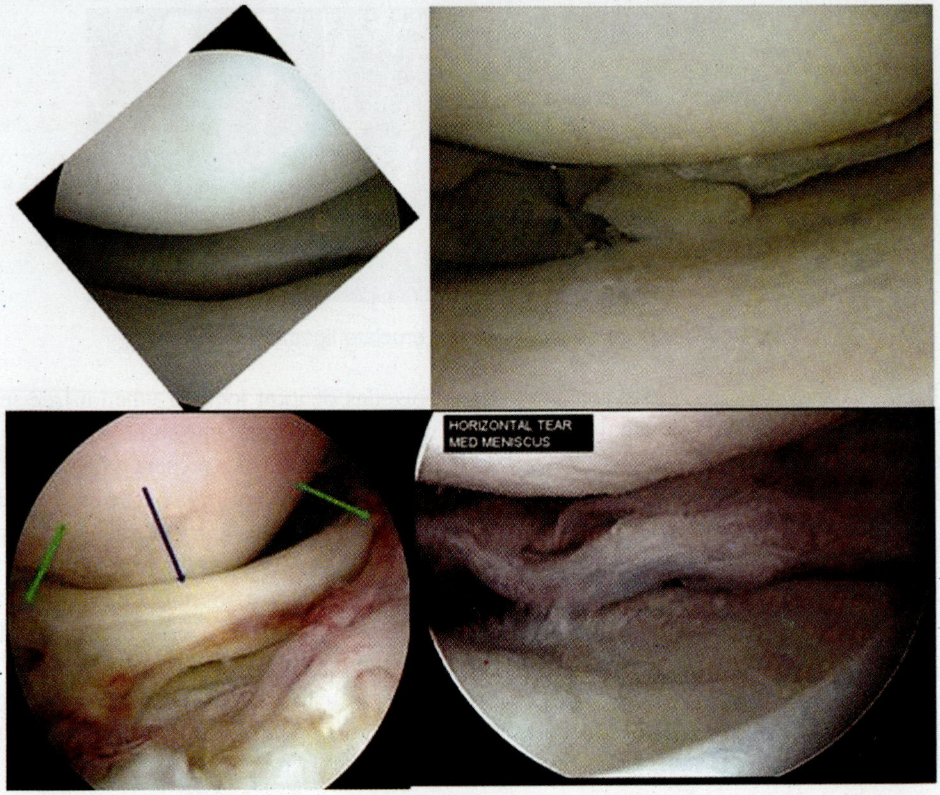

Fig. 11.23: (Top Left) Arthroscopic picture of normal meniscus; (Top Right) Torn meniscus—Parrot beak tear; (Bottom Left) Bucket handle tear of meniscus (arrows) (Bottom Right) Degenerative horizontal tear of meniscus

knee in 90° flexion. Mild rotation of tibia after a period of rest in above position with careful traction along the axis of the leg will usually result in reduction. Persistent symptoms are treated by surgery. Only outer third of meniscus is vascular and tears here are repaired by suturing. All other tears of meniscus are debrided and excised arthroscopically. Menisectomy, however, exposes articular cartilage to much greater forces than normal and leads to earlier onset of osteoarthritis. Associated lesions, such as ACL or PCL tears are treated on their merits.

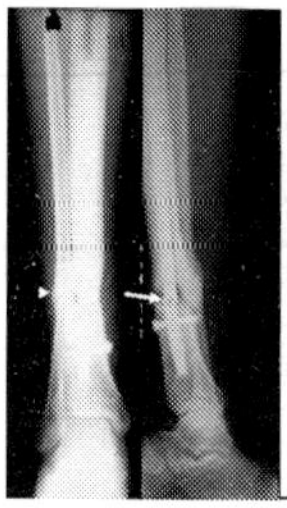

12 Injuries of the Leg, Ankle and Foot

Tibia and fibula, Ankle, Dislocation Ankle, Soft tissue injuries, Tarsal bones, Metatarsal and Phalanges

INJURIES OF THE LEG—FRACTURES OF THE TIBIA AND FIBULA

These are extremely common injuries in all age groups and are frequently open, sometimes with very extensive and contaminated wound. These injuries can occur following road traffic and sports accidents. Though the tibia and fibula most often fracture together (both bones run parallel to each other and are tightly bound together by ligaments), the tibia is the most important consideration as it does most of the weight bearing of the leg and its length and alignment need to be restored as accurately as possible for full function. The fibula is responsible for 6% to 16% of weight bearing and its injuries are relevant only for the three reasons: (a) distally, the fibula is essential for ankle stability; (b) common peroneal nerve winds around the neck of the fibula, and is almost subcutaneous in this region and hence prone to direct blows or traction injuries; and (c) in the fracture of the both bones of the leg, fibula often heals rapidly and may sometimes hold the fracture fragments of (hitherto ununited) tibial fracture apart and prevent union of the tibial fracture.

Mechanism of Injury and Types

Fractures of the both bones of the leg may be caused by direct injury, or indirect injury.

Direct injury is often high energy injury (as in motor vehicle accidents) and leads to transverse, comminuted, displaced fractures. These fractures have high incidence of soft tissue injuries. Indirect injury occurs by twisting injury and leads to spiral, undisplaced fractures with minimal comminution and minimal soft tissue damage.

The fractures of the both bones of the leg can be classified as open versus closed, according to the anatomic location (proximal, middle or distal third), presence or absence of comminution, fracture configuration (transverse, spiral, oblique), displacement (undisplaced versus displaced—percentage of cortical contact) and according to the presence or absence of associated injuries.

Clinical Features

Patient gives history of pain in the leg and inability to ambulate after sustaining a low or high energy injury. The diagnosis is usually obvious on inspection. Deformity, swelling, shortening of the leg and abnormal mobility at the fracture site are indicators of the injury. In addition, color of the extremity for vascular perfusion (pinkish colour indicates good perfusion while gray or dusky colour indicates circulatory compromise). The soft tissues should be carefully evaluated for contusions or breach of skin suggesting compounding. Wounds should be assessed for size, location, degree of contamination and severity of tissue injury. Neurovascular status should be assessed and compartment syndrome should be ruled out.

X-rays: Radiographic evaluation must include entire leg with knee and ankle (anteroposterior and lateral views; oblique views are sometimes necessary to characterize the fracture). The

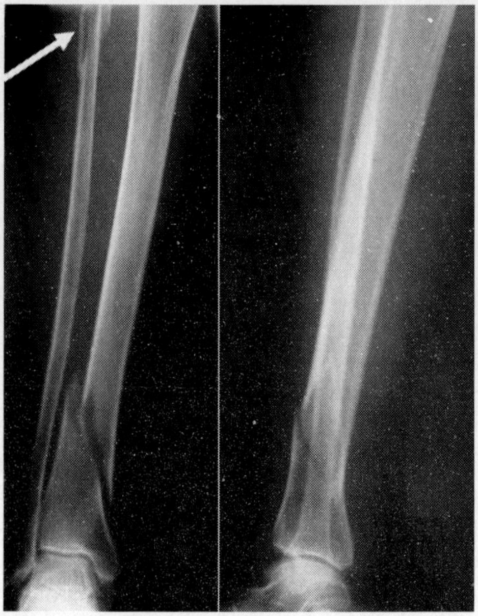

Fig. 12.1: Fracture both bones of the leg. Note that the fibular fracture (arrow) is very proximal in this case. Also note that knee should have been included in these X-rays

location, fragment number and position (comminution, butterfly fragments), fracture configuration, angulation, shortening, displacement (expressed as percentage of cortical contact) and rotation are noted (Fig. 12.1).

Treatment

Nonoperative treatment: Reduction followed by the application of a long-leg cast with progressive weight bearing is the most common method used in the treatment of these fractures (Fig. 12.2).

The criteria for acceptable reduction include:

- Less than 5 degrees of varus/valgus angulation
- Less than 10 degrees of anterior/posterior angulation.
- Less than 10 degrees of rotational deformity (external rotation is tolerated better than internal).
- Less than 1 cm shortening
- More than 50% cortical contact.

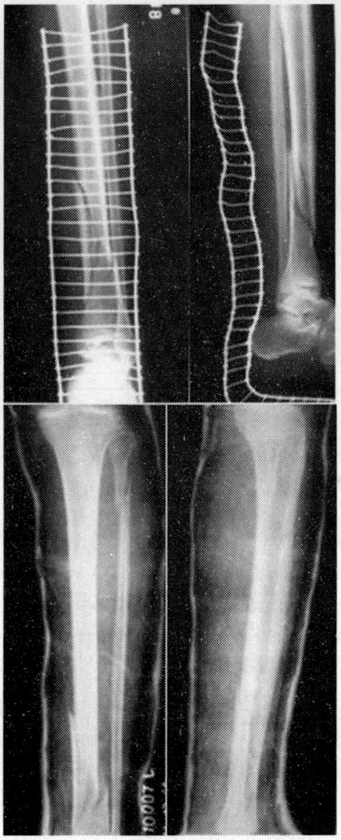

Fig. 12.2: Conservative treatment of both bones leg fracture. (Top) Pre manipulation X-rays. (Bottom) X-rays following manipulation and POP. Note that the reduction is acceptable

The plaster is applied with the knee in 0° to 5° flexion to allow for weight bearing with crutches as soon as tolerated in the minimally displaced fractures. Time taken to union is 16 $\pm$ 4 weeks. X-rays are taken every 6 or 8 weeks to evaluate healing. A patellar tendon bearing (PTB) cast is sometimes applied to allow knee movements after 6 to 8 weeks following injury. Cast brace (functional brace) can be applied (to substitute for full plaster) after four to six weeks of injury with hinges at the knee and optionally at ankle.

Operative treatment is indicated in:

- Most compound fractures (except those with puncture wounds or those without significant soft tissue disruption)

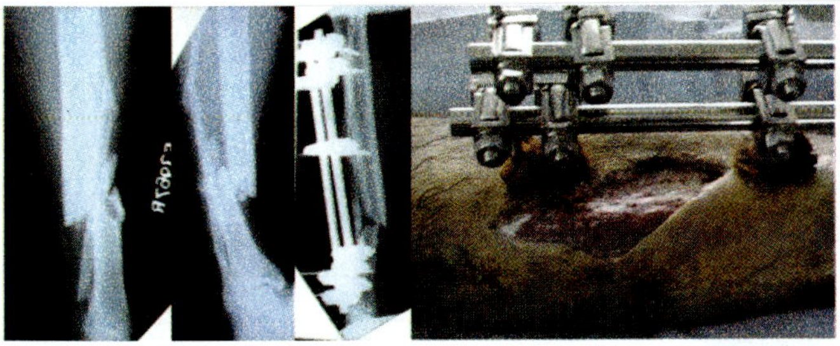

Fig. 12.3A: Compound fracture both bones leg treated by tubular external fixator

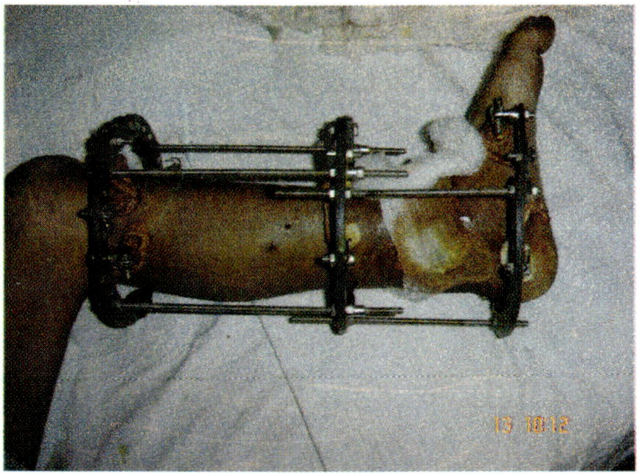

Fig. 12.3B: Compound fractures can also be treated by Ilizarov ring fixator

- Fractures with vascular injury
- Fractures with compartment syndrome
- Fractures with associated ipsilateral femoral shaft fractures. In polytraumatized patient stabilization of tibial fracture improves patient mobility, facilitates nursing, minimizes pain and reduces risk of ARDS.
- Inability to achieve or maintain reduction.

External fixation (Fig.12.3) is primarily used to treat open fractures, fractures in burns patients, fractures in patients with impaired sensations and in closed fractures with compartment syndrome following decompression. It allows easy access to soft tissues and partial weight bearing after wound healing. Delayed healing and non-healing may occur in upto 10% patients. Pin tract infections are common (in 10 to 15% cases).

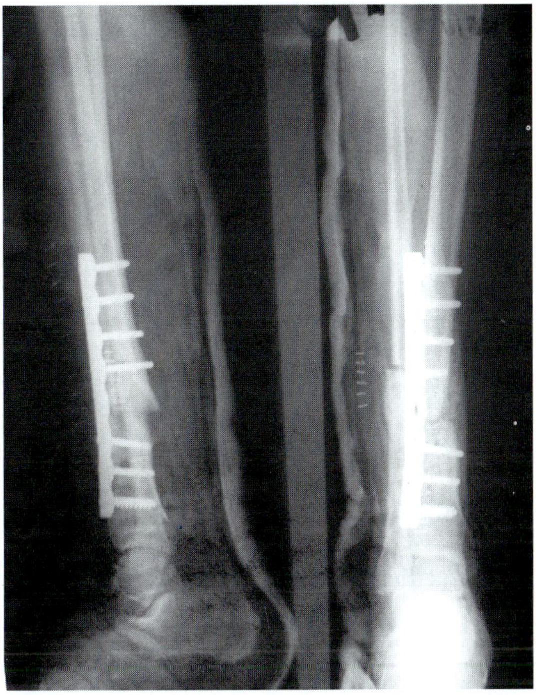

Fig. 12.4: Fracture both bones of leg treated by plating of tibial fracture. Note that the fracture of the fibular shaft can be ignored

Open reduction with internal fixation (ORIF) with plates and screws is generally reserved for fractures extending into metaphysis or epiphysis (Fig. 12.4). Complication include infection, wound breakdown and mal-or non-union.

Intramedullary nailing (Fig. 12.5) preserves soft tissue attachments and blood supply and achieves proper alignment of the fractures. Use

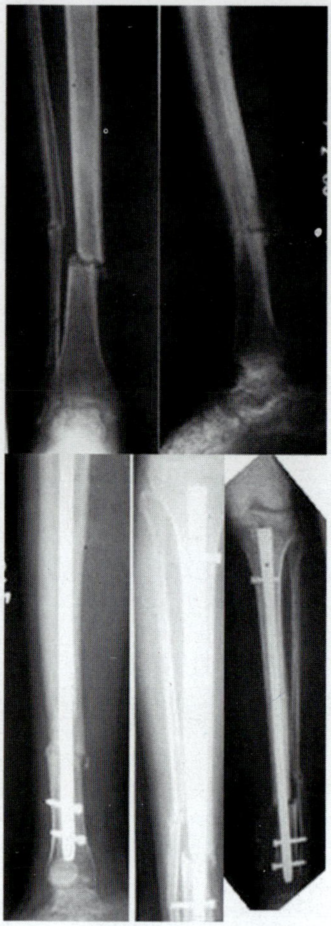

Fig. 12.5: Fracture both bones of leg treated by interlocking nail

of proximal and distal interlocking screws maintains proper length and alignment of even unstable/comminuted fractures until healing has occurred. Disadvantages include the risk of disruption of the endosteal circulation to bone.

Fasciotomy is done when there is evidence of compartment syndrome.

Flap coverage is indicated when there is inadequate soft tissue to cover the bone, tendon, nerves, vessels, and orthopedic implants. Soft tissue defects of the proximal third of the leg can be covered with a medial gastrocnemius muscle flap. Defects of middle third of leg can be covered by soleus flap while defects of the distal third of the leg require free vascularized muscle flap.

Amputation may be optimal treatment for severely crushed leg and foot or open fractures with neurovascular injuries.

Complications

Early: (hours to days)
- Neurovascular injury
- Soft tissue loss
- Compartment syndrome
- Fat embolism

Delayed: (days to weeks)
- Reflex sympathetic dystrophy
- Infection (open fracture/ operated fracture)
- Stiffness at knee and/or ankle
- Claw toes (due to scarring of extensor tendons or ischemia of posterior compartment muscles)

Late:
- Malunion (Fig. 12.6)
- Delayed union

Non union (Fig. 12.7) occurs due to high velocity injuries, open fractures, infection, intact fibula, poor apposition/contact of fracture fragments and inadequate fixation. Treatment is by autogenous iliac crest bone grafting alongwith

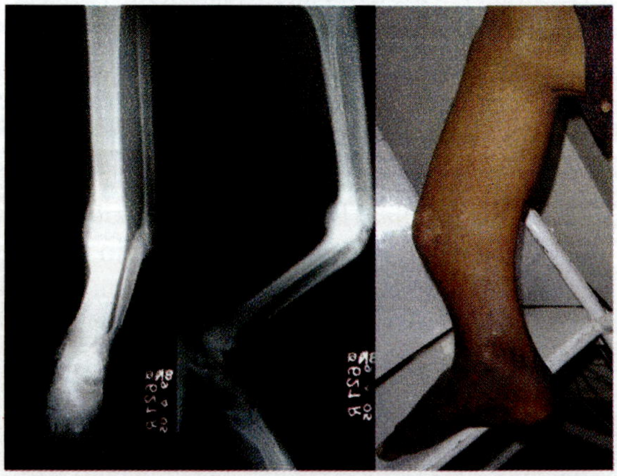

Fig. 12.6: Malunion of both bones leg fracture—X-ray and clinical appearance

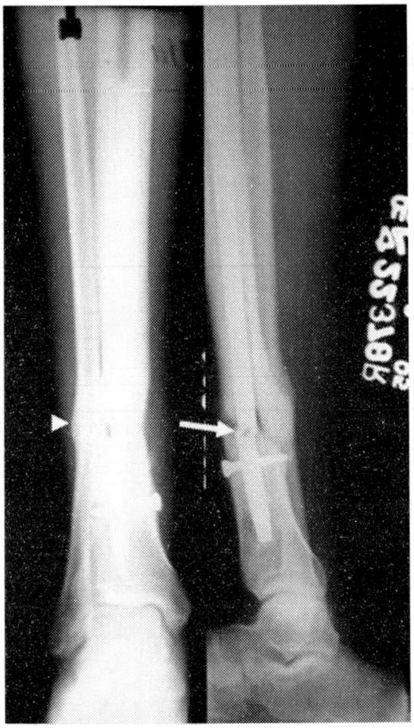

Fig. 12.7: Non union of tibia fracture with interlocking nail *in situ*. Note that the fibula has united (arrow head) and nail has broken at the non union site through the screw hole (long arrow)

internal fixation, revision of inadequate internal fixation, or plaster immobilization.

Fractures of the Tibia Alone

Tibia alone may be fractured leaving fibula intact in direct trauma, twisting injuries (Fig. 12.8) and stress fractures. Stress fractures occur due to repeated, unaccustomed activity seen in military recruits (occur at posteromedial cortex at metaphyseal/diaphyseal junction), ballet dancers (occur in the middle third), hurdlers and long distance runners. In these cases, symptoms may be bilateral, onset of symptoms is insidious, radiographic findings may be delayed for several weeks (X-rays are normal in early course) and bone scan may suggest the diagnosis.

The isolated fractures of tibia are treated the same way as fracture of both bones. Stress fractures require cessation of offending activity. Sometimes in these cases, a short leg cast may be necessary; with partial weight bearing, ambulation can be allowed and fracture heals in 6 to 10 weeks.

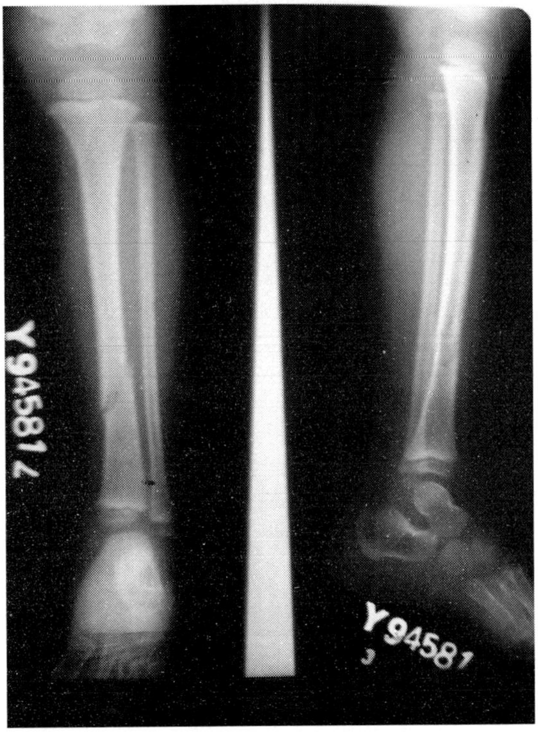

Fig. 12.8: Undisplaced isolated fracture of tibia in a child. These fractures are common in children and result from indirect injury. These are treated conservatively in POP cast.

Isolated Fibular Fractures

Fibula alone can be fractured by direct trauma, twisting injuries and repeated stress in long distance runners. Twisting injuries of particular importance are Maisonneuve fractures where spiral fracture of the upper third of fibula may be associated with fracture of tibia at the ankle. Therefore, ankle must be examined radiologically in every patient with an apparently isolated fracture of fibula (Fig. 12.9), so that a tibial fracture is not missed. Also, these injuries need operative treatment (ORIF using screws and plates). Otherwise, treatment of isolated fibular fracture consists of weight bearing as tolerated. Long leg cast is sometimes required for relief of pain or in stress fractures.

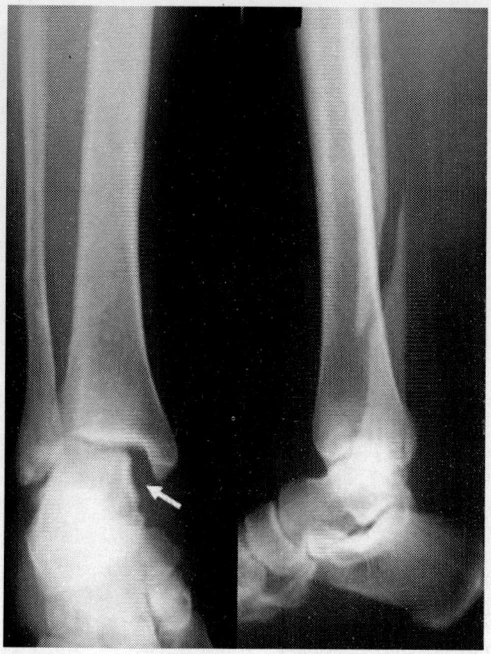

Fig. 12.9: Isolated fracture of fibula may be associated with subluxation of the ankle joint. Note the increased medial space (arrow) due to talar subluxation. A medial (deltoid) ligament injury is associated in this case

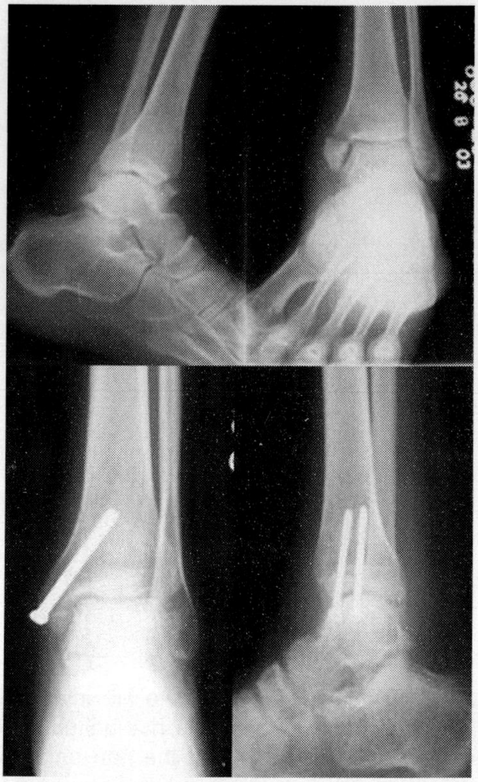

Fig. 12.10: (Top) Transverse fracture of medial malleolus; (Bottom) Fixation by two screws. These fractures are avulsion injuries

INJURIES AROUND ANKLE

Injuries around ankle are common and certain salient features must be kept in mind while treating ankle injuries:

1. Bony injuries and ligament injuries frequently coexist and any treatment plan must include both types of injuries.

   Remember: Bones may be broken in the ankle at 3 points:

   a. Medial malleolus of the tibia.
   b. The lower end of the fibula including lateral malleolus, and
   c. The "posterior malleolus", or posterior margin of the tibia.

   Three ligaments may be torn, namely, the inferior tibio fibular ligament, the medial (deltoid) ligament and the lateral collateral ligament.

   Note: Displaced malleolar fractures are always accompanied by a ligamentous injury (usually on the opposite side e.g. medial malleolar displaced fracture is associated with lateral ligament injury).
2. Transverse malleolar fractures (Fig. 12.10) are avulsion injuries (by attached ligament); vertical malleolar fractures are secondary to impaction by talus.
3. Ankle bears more weight per unit area than any other joint in the body. Any incongruence or malunion leads to traumatic arthritis of ankle due to excessive stresses on joint. For example, a lateral shift of talus by 1 mm will decrease surface contact by 40%.
4. The syndesmosis between distal tibia and fibula may be injured and must be diagnosed and treated precisely.

5. Key to successful management of ankle fractures is distinguishing between the stable and unstable injuries. The bones and ligaments of the ankle essentially form a ring (composed of the tibial plafond, medial malleolus, deltoid ligament, calcaneus, lateral ligaments, lateral malleolus, and interosseous membrane) around the joint (Fig. 12.11). Like the pelvic ring, a single break is a stable injury whereas a ligament injury or fracture on both the medial and lateral sides of the ring leads to unstable injury. Isolated undisplaced fractures of the lateral, medial or posterior malleolus and undisplaced fractures of the distal fibular shaft are stable and can be managed nonoperatively.

Mechanism of Injury and Types

The forces acting on the ankle that result in a fracture are typically combination motions and

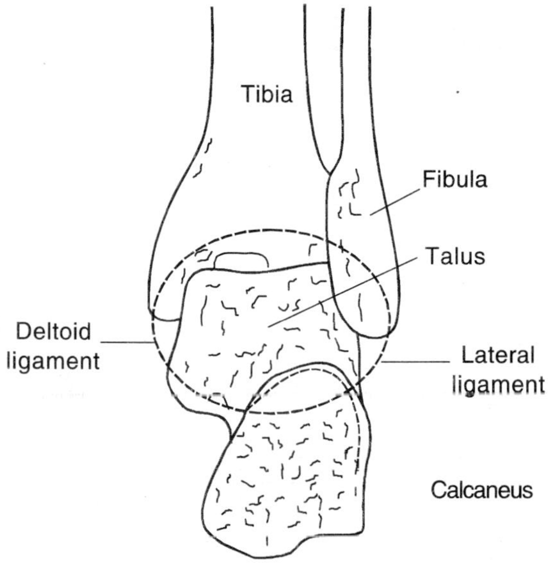

Fig. 12.11: The ring of ankle mortise

patient often only gives history of 'twisting'. The pattern of ankle injury depends on mechanism, age of the patient, bone quality and the position of the foot at the time of injury. Four forces may contribute to injury, namely:

a. Abduction (force which displaces talus laterally)
b. Adduction (force which displaces talus medially)
c. External rotation, and
d. Vertical compression (as in fall from height).

Several complex classifications of ankle fractures are available but it is more useful to know the typical patterns of ankle injury and ligamentous injuries. The ankle fractures involving malleolar projections include: Isolated medial or lateral malleolar fractures, bimalleolar and tri malleolar fractures. Fracture dislocations occur when a fracture of the ankle region is associated with dislocation of the talus out of the ankle mortise.

Clinical Features

Patient presents with the history of a twisting injury or a low-energy fall, local swelling, ecchymosis, occasional deformity, or, rarely, neurovascular compromise.

X-Rays

Anteroposterior, lateral and mortise views of the ankle should be obtained. Anteroposterior X-ray is seen to evaluate the fracture location and configuration, relationship between the tibia and fibula and any tilt of the talus in the ankle mortise.

Lateral view shows congruity of the ankle joint and posterior malleolus fractures.

Mortise view (Anteroposterior X-ray taken with foot in 15 to 20 degrees of internal rotation) shows relationship of the distal tibia with talus (especially any shift or tilt of talus).

- Transverse fractures are caused by avulsion forces and oblique by talar impact against malleoli.
- An oblique medial malleolus fracture after an inversion injury should raise suspicion of an associated lateral ligament sprain (and possibly unstable ankle–2 breaks in ring!).
- An oblique fracture of the distal fibula 2 to 3 inches proximal to the ankle mortise may

be associated with a medial joint injury and disruption of the tibio fibular ligaments.

- Displaced malleolar fractures are usually accompanied by a ligamentous injury on the opposite side of the ankle.
- Recognize unstable ankle fractures
  - Fractures of both medial and lateral malleoli (bimalleolar fractures).
  - Trimalleolar fractures (bimalleolar plus posterior malleolus)
  - Malleolar fracture on one side with an associated ligament disruption on the opposite side.
- Farther (more proximal) the distal fibular fracture line from the joint line, the higher the likelihood of instability because of the medial malleolus or deltoid ligament disruption.

Remember 'Headset sign': the distal tibia sits on the talus like a head piece on its receiver. When properly seated the space between the handle and the cradle is even—when it is not, injury is present.

Treatment

The goal of treatment is to restore the ankle joint anatomically. Therefore, the treatment is based on the amount of distortion of the anatomic structures and articular incongruity. Fibular length and rotation must be restored to obtain an anatomic reduction.

Non operative treatment is indicated for undisplaced stable fractures or displaced fractures where stable anatomic reduction is achieved.

Isolated lateral malleolus fractures can be treated with protected weight bearing in a walking cast or brace. (**Remember:** Only 6% to 16% weight passes through lateral malleolus; and ligament structures and medial stability prevent displacement).

Isolated medial malleolus fractures are treated in a below knee cast and protected weight bearing is allowed after 4 weeks and plaster is continued till 8 weeks.

Open reduction and internal fixation is indicated for the failure to achieve and/or maintain reduction, displaced or unstable fracture with talar dispalcement or widening of the mortise by 2 mm and open fractures. The malleolar fractures are fixed using lag screws or Kirschner wires with tension banding (Figs 12.12A and B). With more proximal fibular injuries, fixation using screws and plates is performed.

After fixation, the limb is placed in a short leg cast and weight bearing is allowed after union, usually following 8-10 weeks.

Complications

1. Soft tissue problems: Such as fracture blisters, swelling, wound necrosis, etc.
2. Non union: Rare, usually involves medial malleolus.
3. Malunion.

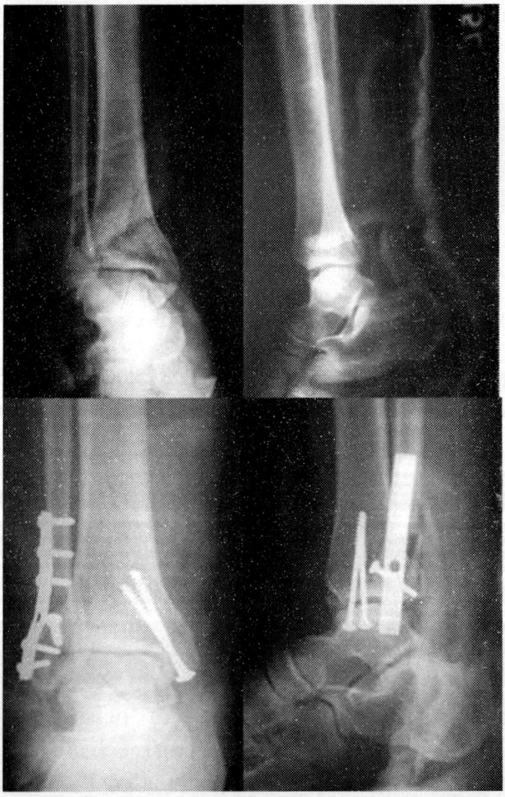

Fig. 12.12A: Bimalleolar fracture fixed by screws for medial malleolus and plating for lateral malleolus

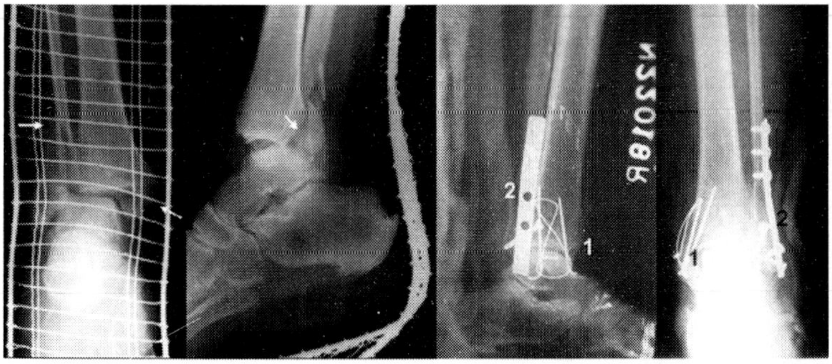

Fig. 12.12B: Trimalleolar fracture. Preoperative and postoperative X-rays. Note the arrows indicating (1) Medial malleolus, (2) Lateral malleolus, and (3) Posterior malleolus fractures. Tension band wiring for medial malleolus and plating for lateral malleolus was done. Posterior malleolus, when small (less than one third articular surface) and reduced, is ignored

4. Post traumatic arthritis.
5. Reflex sympathetic dystrophy.

Ankle Injuries in Children are epiphyseal injuries which can be Type II (Fig. 12.13A) with little potential for growth damage or Type III (Fig. 12.13B) or IV usually seen as fracture of medial malleolus of various types with potential for growth disturbance.

ANKLE DISLOCATIONS AND FRACTURE DISLOCATIONS

Ankle dislocations without fractures are very rare because of the mechanical stability of the mortise and great amount of force required to tear the ligaments. Ankle dislocations are frequently associated with fracture (Fracture-dislocations) (Figs 12.14A and B). The ankle dislocations and fracture dislocations are caused by high energy trauma. Clinically, there is an obvious deformity. There may be compounding or tenting of skin over a fracture fragment. Treatment comprises urgent reduction of ankle to prevent skin necrosis and/or vascular compromise and to relieve pressure on the articular surface. After reduction of the ankle, the fracture component is treated on the lines of treatment of ankle fracture.

SOFT TISSUE INJURIES OF THE ANKLE

Ankle sprain: Ankle sprain is the commonest ligament injury of the human body. Sprain of the ligament occurs due to forced inversion of the ankle which is not severe enough to produce rupture of the lateral ligament. The patient presents with pain and swelling at the ankle and difficulty in walking. The lateral ankle is tender and ecchymotic. Plantar flexion and inversion of the ankle produces severe pain. Radiographs are usually normal. Treatment is immobilization in a below knee POP cast for 3-6 weeks.

Rupture of Tendo Achilles

Tendo achilles rupture occurs commonly but is often missed. In elderly it occurs at insertion of the tendon while in young patient it occurs at the musculo-tendinous junction. The commonest mechanism of injury is forced dorsiflexion of the plantar flexed foot. Patient presents with a history of a snap or 'pop' or of feeling of being hit in the back of the heel. Examination reveals tenderness of the heel cord and a palpable defect. Squeezing the calf does not cause plantar flexion when the patient is lying prone (Thompson's test). Patient is unable to stand on his tip toes. Ultrasound and MRI are diagnostic modalities of choice.

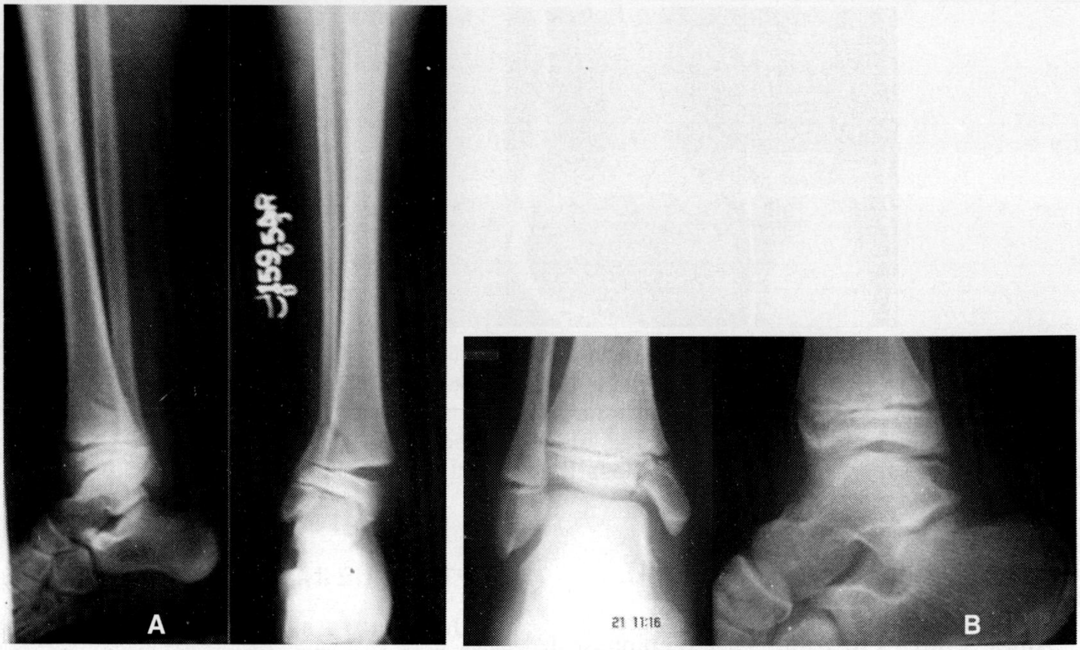

Fig. 12.13: Epiphyseal injuries around ankle. (A) Type II epiphyseal injury without any risk of growth disturbance (B) Type III epiphyseal injury type of medial malleolus fracture

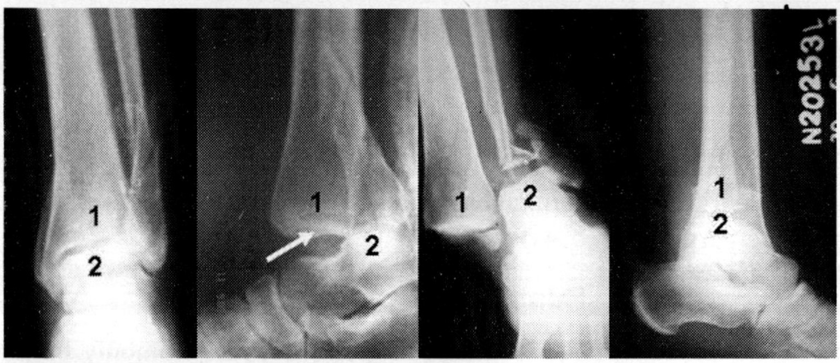

Fig. 12.14A: Fracture dislocation of ankle (Far left and second from left). Note that although AP view looks fine, the lateral view shows loss of contact (arrow) between distal tibia (1) and articular surface of talus (2) alongwith fracture of lower fibula and posterior malleolus. (Right) severe fracture dislocation of ankle in another patient

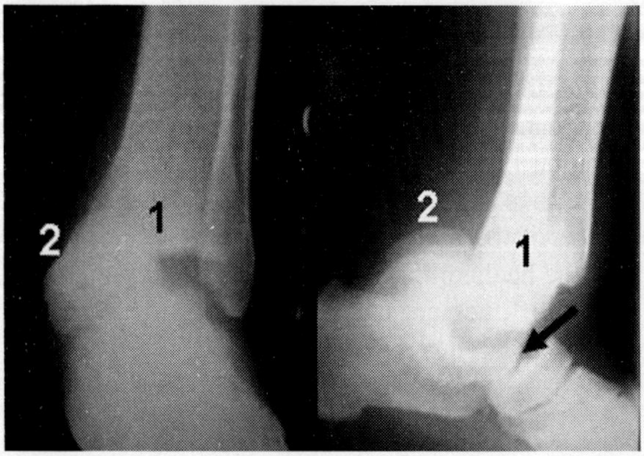

Fig. 12.14B: Dislocation of ankle. Note that talus is no more articulating with tibia or navicular (black arrow)

Treatment

Nonoperative treatment consists of above knee POP cast with flexion at knee and plantar flexion at ankle which is gradually reduced to plantigrade. However, active and athletic patients can be treated by direct operative repair of the tendon followed by protection in POP cast. Complications include wound slough, infection and rerupture of tendon.

INJURIES OF TARSAL BONES

Fractures of Talus

The talus has three parts: the head which articulates with navicular, the neck (non articular), and, the body, which articulates with tibia above and calcaneus below. Talus has no muscular or tendinous attachments therefore its blood supply is tenuous and it is prone to avascular necrosis following injuries.

Mechanism of Injury and Types

Fractures of the talus are caused by high energy injuries as in fall from heights and motor vehicular accidents. Fractures may involve head, neck or body. Talar neck fractures are commonest and are also called *aviator's astragalus* as they occur with forced dorsiflexion as in a plane crash (when foot is jammed against the floorboard).

Clinical Features

Patient presents with swelling, tenderness and pain that may be poorly localized. The pain is aggravated by ankle motion. When associated with dislocation, the fragment (usually proximal), may tent the overlying skin with impending necrosis. Sensations and pulses in the foot should be carefully documented in such cases.

X-rays

AP, lateral and oblique views of the ankle are needed. Fractures of the neck and body are best seen on lateral view (Fig. 12.15) while AP and oblique views are necessary to assess the amount of displacement and the alignment of talus in the ankle mortise. Associated dislocations as well as fractures of malleoli must be looked for. CT scan may be needed sometimes to supplement imaging.

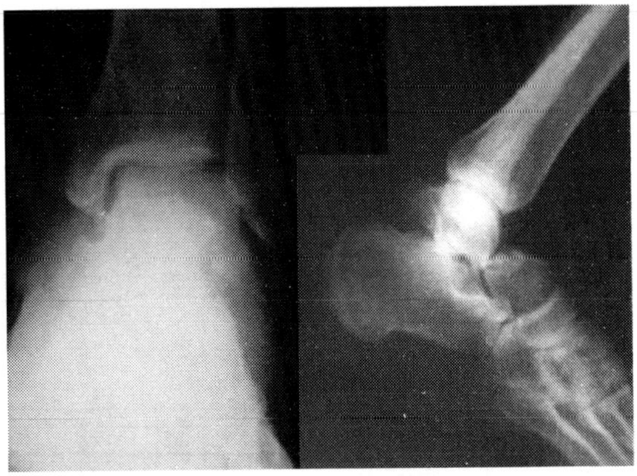

Fig. 12.15: Fracture neck talus. Note that fracture is best seen on lateral view (right)

Treatment

Undisplaced fractures of talus neck are treated in below knee POP cast for 6 weeks without weight bearing followed by 4 to 6 weeks in walking cast till union is documented radiologically. Displaced fractures are treated by urgent closed reduction to avoid skin necrosis or vascular compromise. If it fails, urgent open reduction should be done. After reduction these fractures can be fixed by K wires or screws.

Complications

1. Skin necrosis and infection.
2. Delayed union or non union.
3. Avascular necrosis (Fig. 12.16).
4. Malunion with varus.
5. Painful arthritis of ankle or subtalar joint.

Fractures of the Calcaneus

Calcaneus is the most often fractured tarsal bone, representing 60% of all tarsal fractures.

Mechanism of Injury and Types

Fractures of the calcaneus are caused by a sudden impact to the hind food, most commonly due to

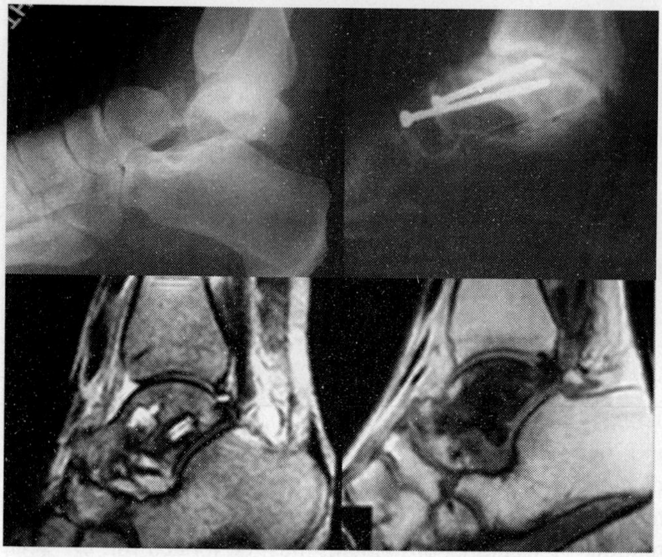

Fig. 12.16: Avascular necrosis of talus (Top) X-rays; (Top left) without treatment. Note that talus looks dense; (Top Right) After screw fixation. Note that the dome of talus is dense and has collapsed. (Bottom) MRI picture of avascular necrosis of talus

fall. Fractures of the opposite side calcaneus and of the dorso lumbar spine should be ruled out in all cases.

Fractures of the calcaneus are classified as intraarticular or extra articular depending on whether the fracture involves the subtalar joint or not (Fig. 12.17). Intraarticular fractures are the commonest and are largely compression fractures.

Clinical Features

Patients with calcaneal fractures present with a widened hind foot with severe pain and swelling. Blistering of overlying skin and compartment syndrome of the foot may be associated. Spine and opposite foot should be clinically examined and neurovascular status must be assessed.

X-Rays

Lateral view of the hindfoot reveals most calcaneal fractures. AP view is not helpful as the other overlying bones obscure the view. Special views such as axial view and Broden's view can demonstrate calcaneal widening and subtalar joint details respectively. All calcaneal fractures must be evaluated with a CT scan.

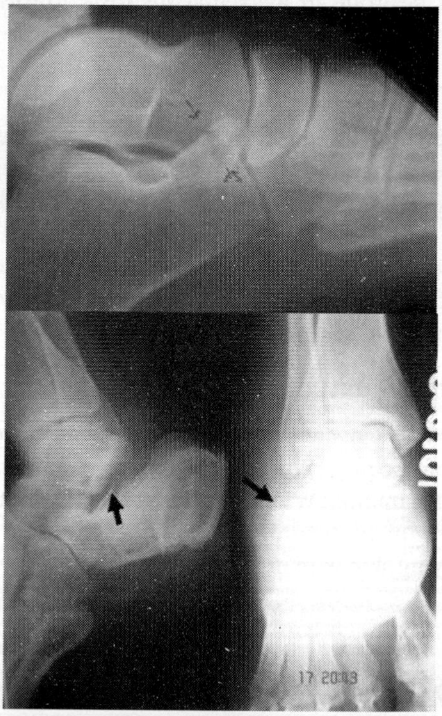

Fig. 12.17: Calcaneal fractures (Top) Extraarticular: Fracture is not involving subtalar joint. (Bottom) Intraarticular fracture. Note on lateral view that articular portion is depressed (arrow). On AP view the lateral wall of calcaneus is blown out (arrow)

Treatment

Fractures without displacement (intraarticular or extra articular) or compression are treated in a below knee cast for 4 weeks.

All compression fractures extending into the subtalar joint, displaced tuberosity fractures (to restore the optimum function of tendo calcaneus) and intraarticular fractures should be surgically treated. Most often open reduction of fracture (and depressed subtalar joint) and fixation with special screws with or without plates alongwith bone grafting is done. Closed reduction and fixation with a spike/Shanz pin may be possible sometimes.

Complications

1. Subtalar stiffness and arthritis.
2. Broadening of heel with peroneal tendon impingement leading to heel pain and inability to wear normal shoes.

FRACTURES OF THE METATARSALS AND PHALANGES

The most common metatarsal fracture is the fracture at the base of the fifth metatarsal (Fig. 12.18). It is caused by sudden inversion of the foot when peroneus brevis tendon avulses its attachment at the fifth metatarsal base. A Jones fracture is a fracture through the proximal metatarsal shaft (Fig. 12.19) which should not be confused with base of fifth metatarsal fracture. The blood supply to this zone is poor and Jones fracture often proceeds to non-union. Ballet dancers may fracture distal fifth metatarsal shaft by landing on it after a jump (Dancer's fracture). The treatment for base of the fifth metatarsal fracture is immobilization in a below knee walking cast for 3 weeks.

Metatarsal shafts may fracture singly or multiply due to a direct blow as due to fall of a heavy object on the foot (Fig. 12.20). Undisplaced fractures or single metatarsal shaft fractures are

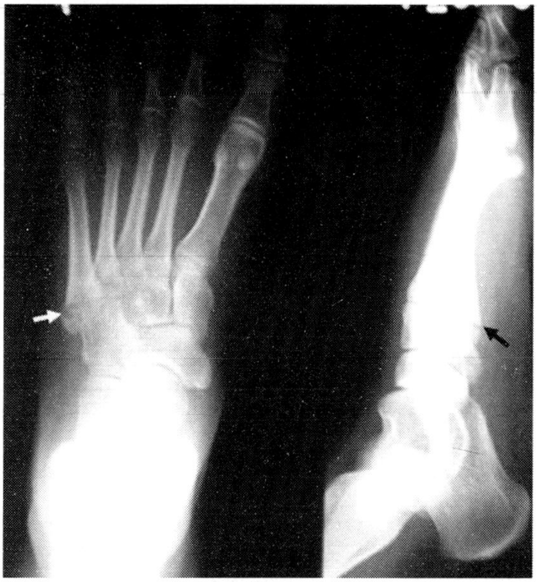

Fig. 12.18: Fracture base of 5th metatarsal. This is an avulsion fracture caused by the pull of peroneus brevis muscle

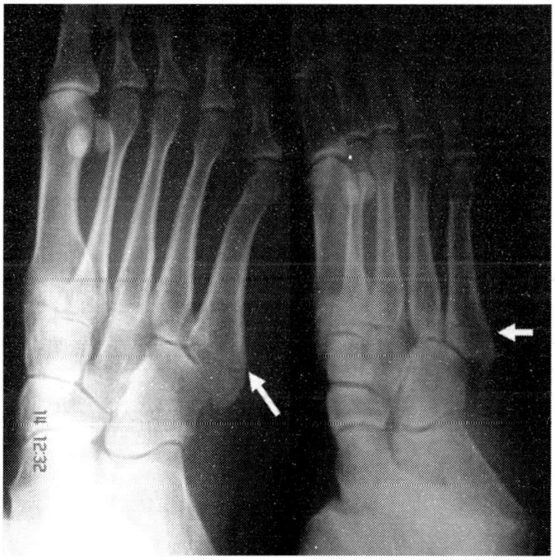

Fig. 12.19: Jones fracture (Proximal shaft of 5th metatarsal)

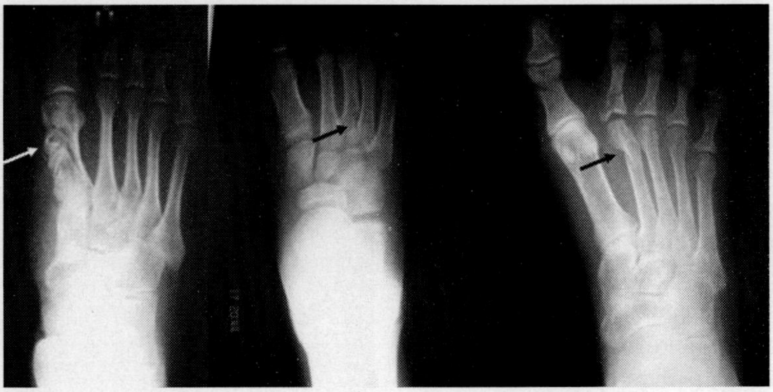

Fig. 12.20: Metatarsal fractures (left) Shaft of first MT (Middle) base of 3rd and 4th MT; (Right) Neck of second metatarsal (Arrows)

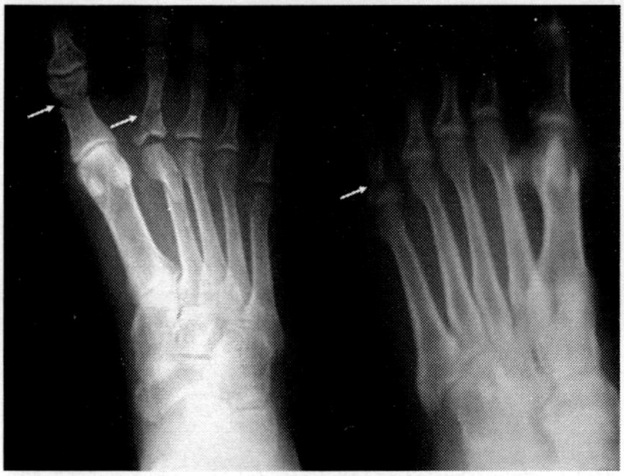

Fig. 12.21: Phalangeal fractures (arrows)

treated in below knee walking cast for 3 weeks. Multiple displaced metatarsal fractures sometimes require surgical fixation (with K wires, screws or small plates) to restore foot stability and alignment.

PHALANGEAL (TOE) FRACTURE (Fig. 12.21)

Toe fractures are caused by direct hit (by stubbing) or due to fall of heavy objects. Most of these can be treated nonoperatively. Buddy splinting (taping the affected toe to adjacent normal one) is effective. Application of a cast to immobilize toe fracture is useless. Patient can be advised to wear hard soled shoe. Rarely, a severely displaced toe fracture or articular injury may need operative pinning.

Glossary

Avascular necrosis	Death of bone from lack of blood supply; osteonecrosis
Aviator's astragalus	Fracture of talus (most often neck) classically caused by plane crash
Avulsion fracture	Fracture of a part of bone which is pulled away by a strong ligamentous or tendinous attachment
Barton's fracture	A fracture of distal radius in which the dorsal or volar articular margin of the radius is displaced
Bennett's fracture	Intrarticular fracture of the base of thumb metacarpal
Boxer's fracture	An impacted fracture of the neck of the fifth metacarpal
Bumper fracture	Fracture of lateral tibial condyle, usually the result of impact on the outer side of knee by car bumper
Burst fracture	A fracture of a vertebral body, usually the result of axial loading, with retropulsion of bony fragments into the spinal canal
Callus	Palpable firm swelling of healing tissue at the fracture site
Chance (Slice) fracture	A fracture of a thoracic or lumbar vertebra, in which the fracture line extends from the spinous process through the pedicles, and then through the vertebral body. An unstable injury, often the result of wearing seat belt
Chauffer's fracture (Backfire fracture or lorry driver's fracture)	Fracture of the radial styloid caused by twisting or snapping injury
Clay Shoveler's fracture	Fracture of the C_7 spinous process
Closed fracture	Fracture does not communicate with the atmosphere (c.f. open fracture)
Colles' fracture	Fracture of distal radius at the corticocancellous junction (within one inch of distal articular surface) with typical (dorsal) displacements. Often seen in post menopausal females following fall on the out stretched hand
Comminuted	Splintered; More than 2 fracture fragments
Compartment syndrome	A syndrome of increased pressure within a tough fibro-osseous compartment due to reduced capacity or increased volume of contents. May jeopardise the viability of muscles within the compartment and the neurovascular structures traversing the compartment.
Complete fracture	Both cortices of the bone are broken.

Compound	The fracture communicates with the atmosphere.
Compression fracture	Fracture caused by axial overload of bone, commonly seen in the spine and calcaneus.
Dashboard injury	Seen in car accidents—posterior dislocation of hip (with or without posterior acetabular lip fracture), femoral shaft fracture, patella fracture, knee ligament(s) injuries—can occur in any combination.
Diastasis	Separation of normally joined parts of slightly moveable joints (syndesmotic joints); occurs in pubic symphysis and distal tibiofibular syndesmosis.
Dinner fork deformity	Typical deformity seen after a malunited Colles' fracture.
Dislocation	A complete disruption of the joint with loss of contact between the articulating surfaces of adjacent bones.
Drawer's test	Test for integrity of cruciate ligaments; Lachman's test also tests ACL
Dunlop traction	A method of skin traction used for treating supracondylar fracutres of the humerus in children.
Essex Lopresti fracture	Fracture of the radial head with disruption of the interosseous membrane leading to proximal migration of radius and disruption of the inferior radioulnar joint.
External fixator	A system of pins drilled into bone and held together by clamps and rods to stabilise a bone or joint.
Fatigue fracture (also "Stress fracture")	Stress fracture occurring due to repeated, unaccustomed (excessive) physical activity in a short period of time in normal bone or chronic stress in a weakened bone.
Floating knee	Fracture of ipsilateral lower femur and upper tibia.
Fracture	Break in the continuity of a bone, epiphyseal plate, or cartilaginous joint surface.
Functional Brace	also called Cast Brace. A brace used for treatment of fractures; uses hydrostatic soft tissue compression to effect and maintain fracture alignment while allowing movements of adjacent joints; especially useful for humerus, tibia fractures.
Galeazzi's fracture-dislocation	Fracture of distal radius with dislocation of inferior radioulnar joint.
Gallow's traction	Skin traction method used for treating femoral shaft fractures in infants and toddlers.
Greenstick fracture	Fracture seen in children where one cortex is fractured and the other is bent but not fractured. Caused by bending force.
Gunstock deformity	Typical deformity after malunited supra condylar fractures of the humerus; contributed largely by cubitus varus.
Hanging Cast	A complete cast applied for the humeral shaft fractures. Often leads to distraction at the fracture and non union because of its weight.

Hangman's fracture	Fracture of the second cervical (C_2) vertebra in which both pedicles are fractured, usually the result of a hyper extension injury.
Hill Sach's lesion (Also called Hatchet Head)	Indentation on (most commonly) posteromedial humeral head caused by the glenoid rim at the time of (mostly anterior) shoulder dislocation. Described in relation to recurrent dislocations (one of the probable causes)
Incomplete fracture	Only one cortex of bone is broken
Jefferson's fracture	Burst fracture of the atlas, usually the result of axial compression
Jones' fracture	A fracture of the proximal diaphysis of the fifth metatarsal
Lisfranc's fracture-dislocation	Fracture dislocation of the tarso metatarsal joint
Malgaigne's fracture	Vertically unstable pelvis fracture with both anterior and posterior fractures in the pelvic ring
Mallet finger (Also called "Baseball finger")	Finger deformity resulting from injury to extensor mechanism; characterised by flexion at DIP joint. May also be caused by fracture or epiphyseal injury of the distal phalanx
Malunion	Fracture healed in a deformed position
Maissonneuve's fracture	Fracture of proximal third of fibula with rupture of distal tibiofibular syndesmosis
March fracture	Stress fracture of metatarsal (most commonly second and third) caused by excessive marching
Monteggia's fracture-dislocation	Fracture of proximal third of ulna with dislocation of the radial head (i.e. dislocation of the proximal radio-ulnar joint)
Non union	The failure of fracture healing to occur
O' Donogue's triad (Unhappy Knee)	Torn anterior cruciate ligament, medial meniscus and medial collateral ligament. Described in American foot ballers
Open fracture	See, compound fracture
ORIF	Open reduction and internal fixation
Osteosynthesis	Operative stabilization of a broken bone with an appliance—plate, nail or external fixator
Pallegrini Steida Disease	Calcification of femoral attachment of medial collateral ligament of the knee after injury
Parry fracture (night-stick fracture)	Isolated fracture of the ulnar shaft, sustained while warding off stick blows
Pathologic fracture	Fracture through diseased bone
Phalen's test	Provocative test for median nerve compression in carpal tunnel. Volar flexion at wrist causes pain.
Pseudoarthrosis	A false joint (due to an ununited fracture)
POP	Plaster of Paris

Pott's fracture	Spiral oblique fracture of distal fibula with associated fracture of medial malleolus or tear of deltoid ligament and lateral displacement of foot on tibia.
PTB cast	Patellar-tendon-bearing cast. A below knee cast moulded around patella, patellar tendon and proximal tibia which allows knee flexion and weight bearing. Used to treat tibial fractures
Reflex dysautonomia	Precipitate rise in blood pressure in quadriplegics and paraplegics in response to noxious stimulus
ROM	Range of motion
Reduce	Set, put into position
Side swipe injury	Comminuted fracture of bones around elbow involving distal humerus, olecranon, shaft of ulna, head of radius and coronoid process
Shenton's line	A smooth curvilinear line tracing medial neck of femur continuing with the inferior margin of superior pubic ramus. A break in the line suggests fracture of femoral neck or dislocated hip
Simple fracture	Fracture with a clean break (without comminution)
Smith's fracture	Reverse Colles' fracture; a distal radius fracture with volar displacement
Spondylolisthesis	Forward slip/displacement of a vertebra on the vertebra below. Hangman's fracture is an example of spondylolisthesis by trauma (C_2 slips over C_3)
Sprain	A torn ligament or joint capsule
Strain	A torn muscle-tendon unit
Straddle fracture	Pelvis fracture with fracture of bilateral superior and inferior pubic rami. Associated with very high incidence of urethral injuries
Subluxation	Partial loss of continuity between the two opposing articular surfaces with some part of the opposing articular surfaces remaining in contact
Teardrop fracture	Avulsion fracture of cervical vertebra where a triangular (tear drop shaped) bony fragment separates from antero inferior vertebral body
Terrible triad of elbow	Elbow dislocation, coronoid process fracture and radial head fracture
Torus (or buckle) fracture	Fracture of only one cortex caused by compressive force seen in children
Triad of vascular injury	Pain, Pallor, Pulselessness
Volkmann's Ischemic Contracture (VIC)	End result of compartment syndrome in which there is contracture, fibrosis and muscle atrophy. Most commonly caused by tight bandage. Supracondylar humerus fracture is the next commonest cause
Volkmann's sign	Sign of contracture of flexor muscles of forearm due to VIC. Extension at wrist causes flexion of fingers (which cannot be extended) while the flexion at wrist allows passive extension of fingers
Wedge fracture	Anterior compression fracture of any vertebra-anterior height becomes less than posterior height. Most common in dorsal spine

Index

F

S

T

V

W